ABANDONED DANSVILLE

THE CASTLE ON THE HILL

BRIAN CRAY

AMERICA THROUGH TIME®
ADDING COLOR TO AMERICAN HISTORY

For my wife, Kelly Cray, and her aunt, Monique Landry,
without your help and support this would have not been possible

America Through Time is an imprint of Fonthill Media LLC
www.through-time.com
office@through-time.com

Published by Arcadia Publishing by arrangement with Fonthill Media LLC
For all general information, please contact Arcadia Publishing:
Telephone: 843-853-2070
Fax: 843-853-0044
E-mail: sales@arcadiapublishing.com
For customer service and orders:
Toll-Free 1-888-313-2665

www.arcadiapublishing.com

First published 2019

ISBN 978-1-63499-154-4

Typeset in Trade Gothic 10pt on 15pt
Printed and bound in England

CONTENTS

1 The Castle on the Hill **5**

2 The Jackson Reign **12**

3 Daily Life **46**

4 The Lion's Roar **49**

5 Quacks, Charlatans, or Business Prodigies? **83**

Endnotes **120**

Bibliography **125**

1

THE CASTLE ON THE HILL

A Brief History

Dansville, named after early settler, Daniel Faulkner, is a small village in Livingston County, New York. In 2010 the population was 4,719 people according to the census, and as of 2016 it is estimated to have decreased to 4,510 people.[1] Dansville, covering only an area of 2.4 square miles, was a hindrance to the Delaware, Lackawanna & Western Railroad for eighty-one years because of the "Dansville Hill," before its mainline abandonment in 1963.[2] However, despite the drawbacks for the railroad, this site became a valuable cornerstone throughout history.

The building on the east hill holds much history in its bare walls, even after thirty-eight years of abandonment. The red façade caked with rusty wrought-iron balconies, evenly spaced among arched crumbling brick windows, still towers six stories high, overlooking the town of Dansville as the "Castle on the Hill." Over a hundred years ago, back in its prime, it employed 255 people, contributed ten percent of tax revenues to the town, and supported a school of nurses, and all this attributed to the fifty-nine-year reign under the Jackson family.[3] In addition to being one of the largest hydrotherapy institutes in the mid-nineteenth century, it was the birthplace of the world's first breakfast cereal and the origin of physical culture, while Dansville became the home to the nation's first Red Cross.

Founded in 1854 by Nathaniel Bingham, a sickly businessman from Rochester, the Castle on the Hill was originally known as the Dansville Water Cure and was first used as a medical facility to scientifically treat and recuperate the invalid.[4] Water cure and the use of the temperate climate, natural springs, and mineralized waters contributed to tackling chronic illnesses in a recreational resort setting. Water cure,

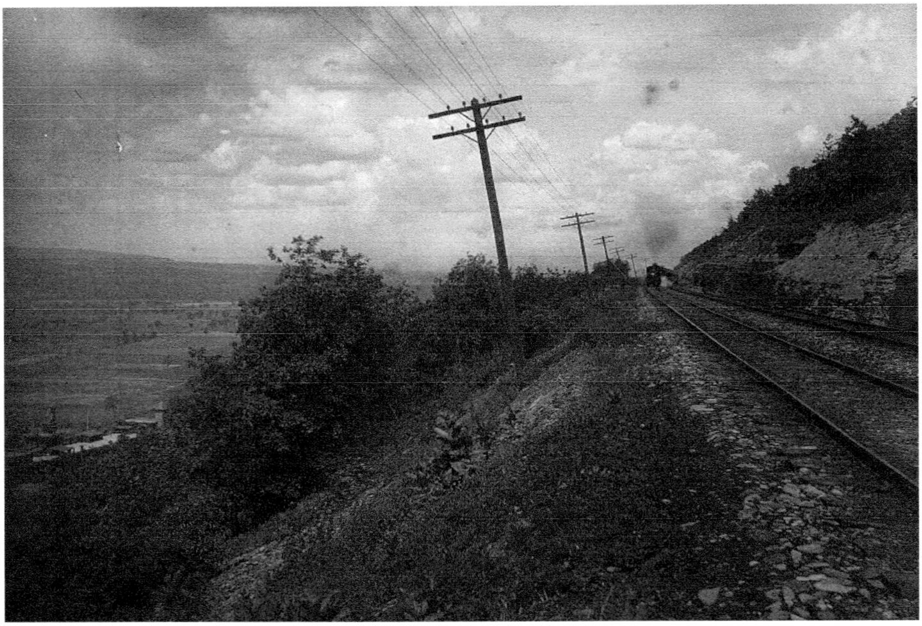

This is the Delaware, Lackawanna & Western Railroad approaching the bend on the Dansville Hill with the castle on the left. The Wayland Train accident in 1943 was one of the worst train wrecks in history, with twenty-six fatalities and multiple injuries. ("26 Killed When Fast Train," 1943) *[Photo by Detroit Publishing Co.]*

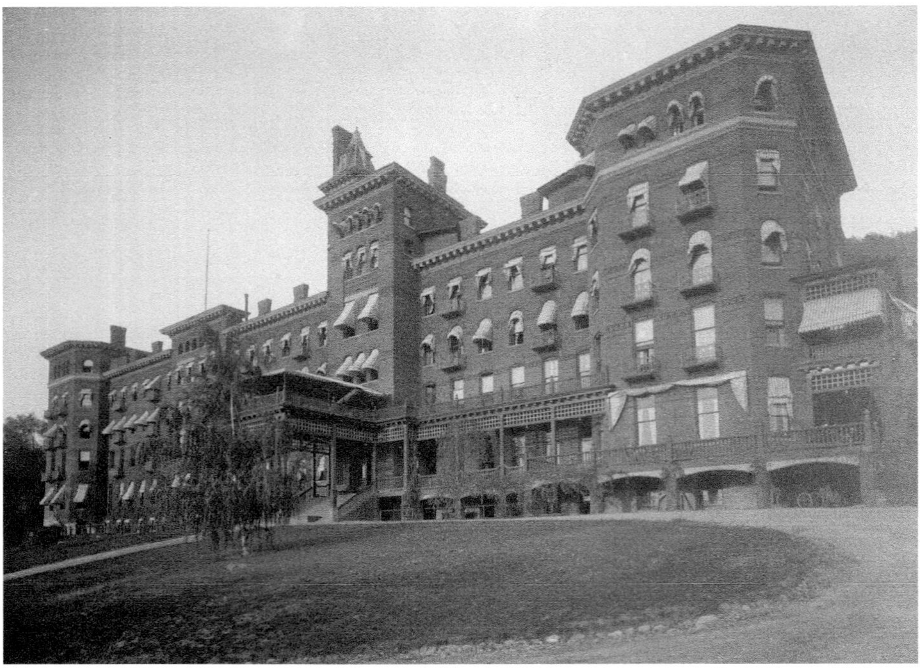

The Jackson Health Resort in its heyday when the wooden balustrade to the patio still wrapped around the façade and the entrance canopy draped over the stairwell serving as a deck to guests. The founder of the resort, Dr. James C. Jackson, became famous from his intellect of novel therapeutics of that era, which we would now consider the application of cult medicine. *[Photo by Detroit Publishing Co.]*

also known as hydrotherapy, was a prevalent method of antiquated cult medicine in the mid-nineteenth century.[5] Its practices originated in Germany and focused on pure water being the alchemy to a life of healthy longevity.[6] Patients undergoing hydrotherapy treatments would endure several baths, showers, douching (cold water shocking), and wet sheet wrappings, as well as drink high quantities of water.[7] Water cure facilities started popping up all throughout America during the mid-nineteenth century and the Dansville Water Cure was one of over 200 hydrotherapy operations across the United States. Alas, after three failed attempts in four years, it closed its doors due to poor leadership.[8]

In October 1858, the castle changed hands when Dr. James Caleb Jackson and his associates, Dr. Hurd and Harriet Austin, took over, changing its name to "Our Home on the Hillside," transitioning eleven years of water cure practice from Glen Haven to Dansville.[9] Jackson was never "officially" owner during his reign, only taking the title of an employee throughout his term as physician-in-chief, but to everyone who knew him or of him, he was the glue, the driving force of the operation. Jackson's water cure helped rehabilitate and soothe patients from nervous breakdowns, but "Our Home" also acted as a diet cure and a facility where the invalid could get well.[10] Tea, red meats, coffee, sugar, alcohol, and tobacco were prohibited there. Jackson focused on a strict regimen consisting of exercise along with a healthy diet of fruits, vegetables, and unprocessed grains, which he coined as "Granula."[11]

Nearing the end of the 1870s, with Dr. James Caleb Jackson's health deteriorating, he stepped down from his position and handed over his responsibilities to his son, Dr. James H. Jackson, and daughter-in-law, Dr. Kate J. Jackson.[12] Duties ran smoothly for a few years up until June of 1882 when a fire broke out from an overturned oil lantern, completely obliterating the main building. Many thought the building met its demise, but months later in October of 1883, the Jackson's opened a new, iron and brick, castle-like structure, deemed "absolutely fireproof." The new building was designed by architect A. J. Warner and cost the Jackson's $200,000, putting operations back to normal in no time, which lasted until 1914.[13] However, with the advancements in pharmacology and science, the philosophy of hydrotherapy flopped, and the Jackson Health Resort declared bankruptcy.[14]

In the years after the Jackson reign, the Army utilized the premises as a psychiatric hospital for World War I Veterans suffering from PTSD.[15] It was not until 1929 that the facility resurrected a new life in the hands of a health enthusiast, Bernarr Macfadden.[16]

When Bernarr purchased the sanatorium, he was sixty-one years old and a health nut, with a highly active daily regimen of exercise and zero interest in slowing down. He was on his fourth wife and had eight kids, but kept much of his personal life a secret.[17] Macfadden was a proponent for the early culture of body building and

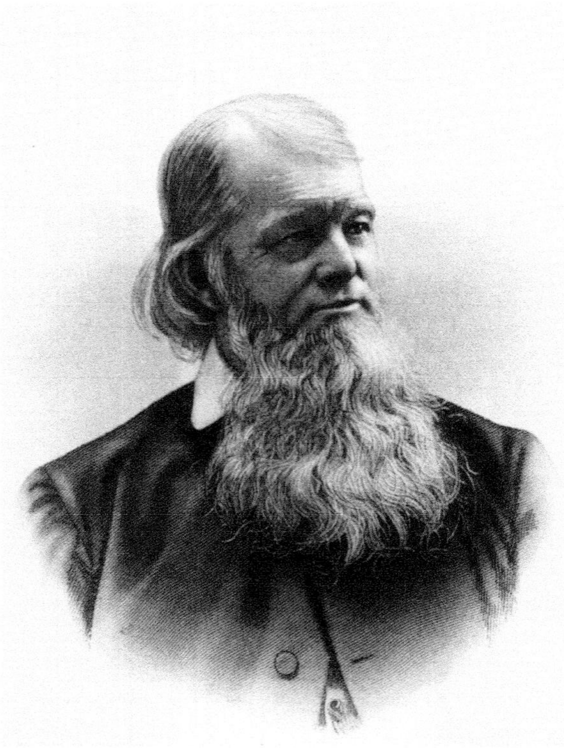

Left: The founder of "Our Home on the Hillside" also known as the "Jackson Sanatorium," Dr. James C. Jackson spent much of his life as a practitioner of cult medicine and as an advocate for diet, health and hygiene. *[Photo by Emily Sartain, National Library of Medicine]*

Below: "Macfadden lived an interesting life of many professions. He was a penniless orphan turned millionaire, a newspaper, magazine and health novel publisher, an author, a school owner, convicted criminal for publishing obscenities, advocate for vegetarianism, sanatorium owner, restaurant owner, champion wrestler, skydiver, circus acrobat, tramp farmhand, dentist's assistant, bookkeeper, clerk, diet specialist and much more!" (Wood, 2010) *[Photo by Bain News Service]*

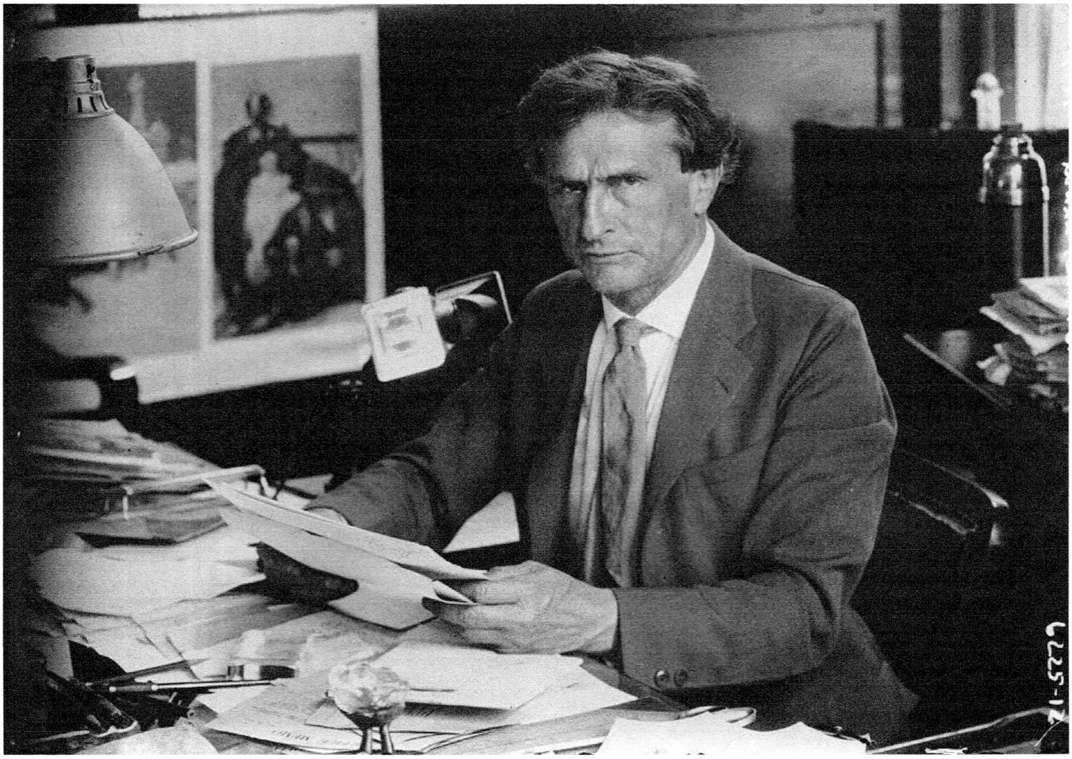

the king behind a publishing empire. He gained much notoriety from his magazine *Physical Culture.*[18] Bernarr renamed the sanatorium to the Physical Culture Hotel. His hotel sponsored multiple events to clench publicity throughout the area, with annual "Cracked Wheat Derbies" consisting of marathons reaching as far away as New York City, promoting the very cereal which runners consumed over two weeks.[19]

Although the P. C. (the nickname of the Physical Culture Hotel) no longer thrived as a water cure facility, it regained much of its prestige through its range of physical recreational activities deemed "therapeutic."[20] Top-notch accommodations for a moderate price, among rumors of the rich and famous, made the P. C. a popular buzz among wealthy patrons, health seekers and vacationers.[21] Among other entertainment, almost every evening included lectures, dancing, card parties, singing, amateur theatricals or even complete programs, where patrons, employees, or reputable artists contributed to the fun. Dancing on the rooftop by its gardens under the starlit sky and sunbathing during the day in the towers made the P. C. the purported place for celebrities to "get away from it all."[22]

However, the unconfirmed rumors of celebrities may have just been a ploy by Bernarr to gain publicity; after all, on his eighty-third birthday he skydived merely to demonstrate the up sides to healthy physical fitness as a publicity stunt.[23]

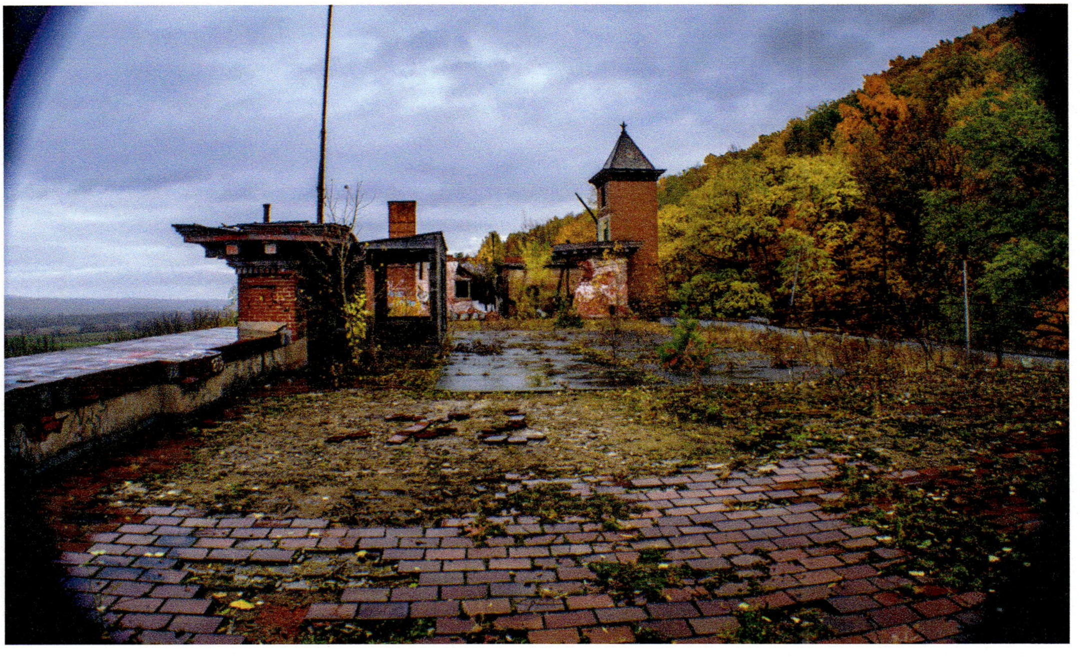

Deep forest camouflages the land below as it encroaches on the rooftop and soon it will take back its dominion as the castle falls further into disrepair and instability. *[Photo by Brian Cray]*

Regardless, he operated the health resort as a successful business venture up until the last three years of his life—He died in 1955.[24] Many believed he died a penniless man, experiencing much financial and legal troubles the last years of his life.[25] His wife at the time, Johnnie Lee Macfadden, claimed otherwise, saying he buried money at multiple locations across the U.S.A., but the only money found was on property he owned in Long Island, when a steel box containing $89,000 was recovered in 1960.[26] Maybe his unearthed personal fortune remains buried somewhere, like the hidden treasures of Lost Dutchman's Gold Mine.

After Macfadden's death, William Fromcheck, a hotelier from New York City, acquired the facility and operated it under the name Bernarr Macfadden's Castle on the Hill.[27] Without the heavy focus on publicity stunts from Bernarr, and his

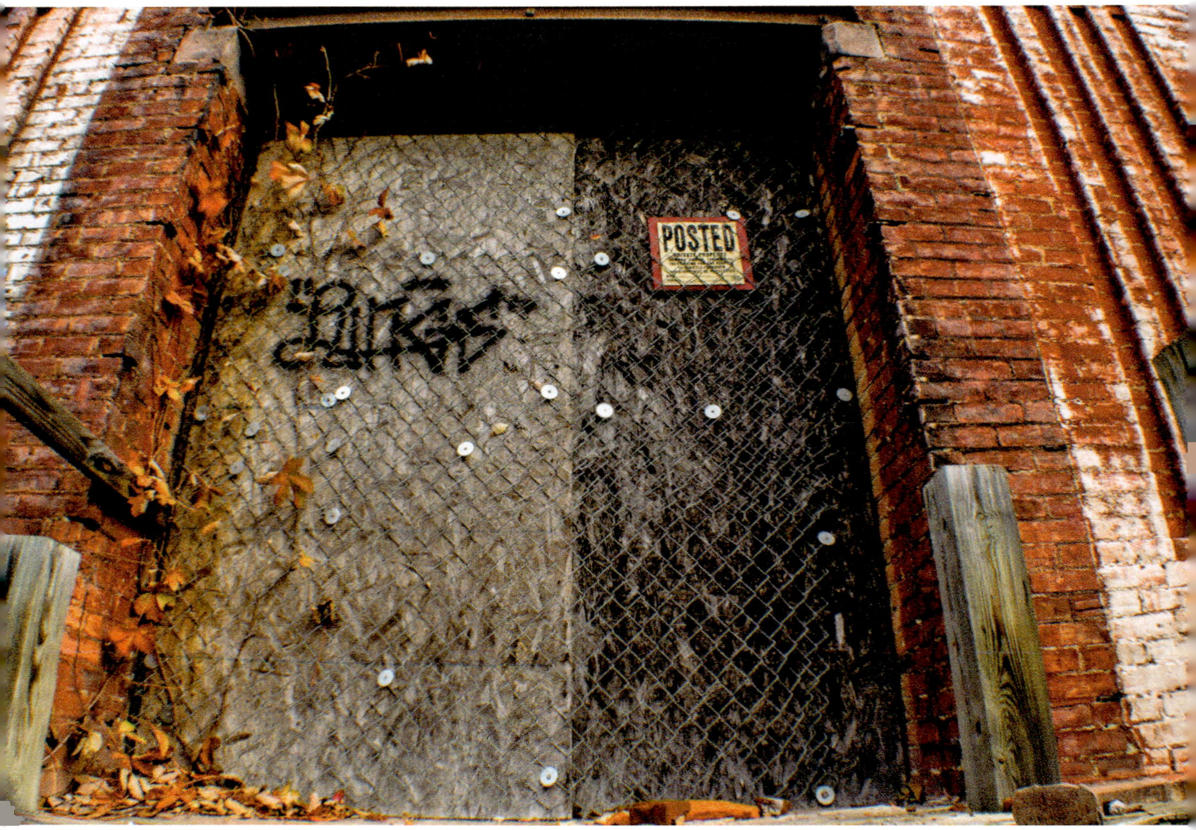

"No Trespassing" signs mark the boarded front entrance to the "Jackson Sanatorium," but that does not stop trespassers in their pursuit to witness beautiful decay despite the steep fines and precarious conditions. *[Photo by Brian Cray]*

prodigious, eccentric personality, the hype around the health spa faded until it finally flopped in 1971.[28] From 1972 to 1978, the building remained vacant with legal impediments from Fromcheck's death occupying the estate. In the meantime, the Bernarr McFadden Foundation searched for potential buyers, and despite all the rumors, it was not until 1978 when a group, Christians Concerned for Human Needs, purchased the estate for $100,000.[29] They changed its name to the Dansville Institute and only kept it running until 1981, when it closed for the last time.[30]

2

THE JACKSON REIGN

A Brief History on James Caleb Jackson and the Leading Water Cure Institute in the World During the Nineteenth Century

BOOM … a loud burst pierced the air like rolling thunder, startling the early settlers of Dansville back in 1798. They scurried up the eastern hillside, wandering up the slippery banks to discover "Breakout Creek," a new stream, and coined the miracle "All Healing Spring." Its herculean force fractured the earth with such strength that it threw 200 to 300 pound rocks down the hillside, among other things, chucking an oak tree clear out of the ground.[1] Its widest fissure, Devil's Hole, went down into the earth over 44 feet.[2] This is where it all began. This phenomenon gave rise to the sanatorium, which would have ceased to exist otherwise. Jackson used the healing properties of the spring to operate one of the most successful hydrotherapeutic institutes of its time.

James Caleb Jackson, born on March 28, 1811, in Manlius, Onondaga County, New York, followed his father's aspiration for him to practice medicine, which came with unduly hard work and discipline throughout his youth.[3] James, at just twelve years old, had already mastered Latin and Greek, completing his education in Troy, New York, at the polytechnic institute. By the age of nineteen, he married Lucretia Edgerton Brewster.

Jackson, having spent the first years of his marriage on a farm in Mexico, New York, dug into the field of medicine because of his deteriorating health and never made it as a farmer.[4] His strong stance as an avid abolitionist fueled his public voice and as the issue of slavery began to bludgeon the nation, he spoke freely within the community.[5] Jackson held many titles over the next ten to fifteen years with his involvement as an agent in the anti-slavery movements in New York and in Massachusetts, and acted as an editor of reformatory papers for the *Madison County Abolitionist, The Albany Patriot*, and staff for *The Emancipator*.[6, 7] His lectures around Oswego County would coin him the title, "Farmer Boy Speaker."[8] He also became highly involved in the state as a public debater, orator, and supporter of women's equality, but in 1846 or 1847, due to his deteriorating health, he relocated to his hometown of Peterboro, New York, and gave up his duties as a full-time abolitionist.[9, 10]

Jackson always suffered from some ailment or health problem, spending much of his life fighting dyspepsia, but in 1847 he latched onto grim death, not expecting to live. With every treatment failing, Jackson placed himself under Dr. Silas O. Gleason's care, which involved his first experiences with hydrotherapy at Glenwood Springs in Cuba, New York. Under Gleason's care, Jackson gave up "coffee and fat sausages" and as a result his health improved drastically like the rebirth of a Phoenix from its ashes.[11] He watched a woman unbelievably recover to full health without the administration of medicine, which left a lasting impression on him. From that day forward, hydrotherapy gave him renewed purpose along with the influence of Sylvester Graham's book, *Science of Human Life*.[12]

He formed a partnership with his wife, with Dr. and Mrs. Gleason, and Miss Theodosia Gilbert, practicing the methods of water cure taught by Priessnitz, a German hydrotherapist. The group opened a water cure facility in Glen Haven along Skaneateles Lake. They adopted Priessnitz's principles of cold-douching (dropping wet rags 16 to 18 ft. upon the ill patients) along with having them drink copious amounts of water "up to twenty to thirty glasses a day."[13] On top of tackling the business affairs of the company, Jackson also attended the Central Medical College of New York in Syracuse, earning his medical degree to fulfill his father's wish while maintaining his prominent voice in woman's suffrage for the NDRA, the National Dress Reform Association.[14, 15]

After just three years, in 1850, Gleason withdrew from Glen Haven Water Cure (The Glen) along with thirty of his patients, leaving Jackson to pick up the slack.[16] Business looked unpromising at first until Jackson cured a teacher of brain fever and patients started piling into The Glen. He capitalized on this by sending an agent to New York to advertise his water cure facility by distributing brochure copies of *The Water Cure Journal*. From this, Jackson planned a hygienic festival in which over 150 people attended The Glen for dinner.[17] His business savvy and leadership made the Glen quite successful and patients visited in droves for treatment without medicine, but Miss Gilbert's (Mrs. Chaplin) death complicated business. She bestowed her inheritance upon her husband, Mr. Chaplin, complicating the future direction of The Glen as he took over her position. Outstanding debts from a fire that broke out in 1854, which eradicated the main building, also complicated matters, and so Jackson took his interests elsewhere.[18]

In 1858, he relocated to Dansville, along with some of his staff, Dr. Harriet Austin, F. Wilson Hurd, and Jackson's two sons, who moved back from Nebraska.[19] He founded Our Home on the Hillside, later known as the Jackson Sanatorium.[20] October 1, 1858, became known as "Founder's Day" marking its opening to the public, which he directed on two principles:

1. Restoring sick patrons to full health
2. Extending his and the institution's philosophies of health through proper living[21]

Jackson felt that teaching the laws of health and rightful living, if employed correctly, would far exceed any administration of drugs.[22] He innovated much of modern mental therapeutics through his "psycho-hygienic" philosophies. He used these principles to treat over 20,000 patients in twenty years at the sanatorium and according to his book, *The Sexual Organism, And Its Healthful Management,* it was "without ever giving any of them any medicine."[23] He believed drugs prescribed to patients by other doctors a fallacy in practice and thus referred to their usage as "poisonous medicines."[24] Through his beliefs and practices the institution grew large enough to accommodate 250 guests, where invalids could bask in the simple life with a surplus of sunshine, the purest of water and salubrious air, and all while living free from the crux of society's fashionable decadent trends and debilitating habits.[25] Guests were free to wear what they pleased at the spa, although Jackson did flaunt the health benefits of wearing the American Costume, which was a revitalized Bloomer.[26]

Jackson believed, "God's mightiest things are his simplest things and nature as a mistress is gentle and holy, and to obey her is to live."[27] His simplistic philosophies became the *Laws of Life*, making him a prestigious figure of Dansville. From his intellect and novel therapeutics, he garnered much success from his skill and application of alternative medicines. He described it as "bringing the whole mind—body, soul, and spirit—into the right relationship to the Divine plan for human life on earth."[28] He believed in the power of mind over matter. Over the span of thirty-six years, *Laws of Life,* a magazine distributed by Jackson and his managerial staff to tens of thousands of subscribers worldwide, indoctrinated their ideologies and philosophies surrounding health and disease, and ultimately centralized these two factors around the preservation of life.[29]

People started to toil with digestion processes as early as the seventeenth century and the fad of vitamins led to entrepreneurial adaptations, as well as quackery within the fledgling field of nutrition.[30] Whether society deemed Jackson a pedantic quack or a miracle worker, that does not quash his success surrounding nutrition and health, much of which he fostered from the preceding principles of Sylvester Graham, one of the first pioneers of vegetarianism in America.[31] Jackson acquired much success through tweaking Graham's beliefs, which focused on a strict regimen of healthier, nonmeat alternatives like vegetables, nuts, roots, seeds, and fruits along with a lower daily caloric intake.[32]

Unlike Graham, who ceased to gain huge financial success from his philosophies (maybe due to his falsifying an MD), during his short lifespan of fifty-seven years, Jackson not only profited from Graham's flour, but stumbled upon the creation of the world's first breakfast cereal in 1863, "Granula," giving him even more international recognition, prestige, and financial triumph among his followers.[33] This fiber-based breakfast alternative to pork and beef did not last, due to its lackluster taste and tedious preparations. It consisted of a two-step baking process. First, Graham flour and a water mixture were baked in a brick oven, followed by grinding the coarse nuggets and re-baking them slowly before soaking the dense bran overnight to make the grains chewable. Often the desired method to serve Granula involved filling one-third of a glass full of the Granula bits and soaking it overnight in the icebox with milk, making it ready for morning.[34] Jackson created Our Home Granula Company, which manufactured Granula and Somo, a healthy coffee that accompanied the breakfast cereal.[35] His creation of Granula would soon trigger the *Cornflake Crusade*, revolutionizing morning meals for years to come as the Kellogg's would master the art of the breakfast cereal in Battle Creek, Michigan.[36] Today, it is a multi-billion dollar industry, all thanks to Dr. Jackson.

Jackson's principles of health-infused hydrotherapy practices focusing on the Graham Plan and abstaining from "poisonous medicines" and vaccinations would go on to influence the foundation of the Battle Creek Sanitarium, led by the first Seventh Day Adventist's.[37]Joshua Himes, Ellen White, and John Kellogg all participated at one time or another in the festivities of Our Home on the Hillside, taking their clever intellect westward and arranging Jackson to deliver lectures demonstrating his expertise, which was not esoteric to their patients.[38] White, upon visiting the sanatorium to take notes on Dr. Jackson's practices to help treat her sick children, adopted a similar dress for the women of Battle Creek, which was not too long, nor too short, and imitated the pattern of the American Costume, charging patrons a dollar per outfit.[39]

After James Caleb Jackson retired in 1879, two generations of Jacksons followed on in the family business, despite a devastating fire burning a majority of the main building and accounting for $40,000 in damages on June 26, 1882.[40] The town invoked Dansville's firefighters and locals to help mitigate the fire that night and all 280 patients fled unscathed, but many thought the building met its demise.[41] However, the rebuild of the castle blanketed its steel frame in red bricks, making it "absolutely fireproof." The operations reopened quickly and up until the following year, Dr. Jackson held an active role in the sanatorium, holding lectures in the chapel and counseling patients with other physicians.

In the years following James Caleb Jackson's death, the Jackson Sanatorium changed names to the Jackson Health Resort, continued leadership under James H. Jackson, and ran under the same principles instilled by the eccentric pioneer of psycho-hygienic philosophies some sixty-nine years prior. The once Spartan practices of the 1860s changed gradually over time as the medical profession began to accept more of the alternative principles backed by the San. Meat was added to the menu, along with more comfortable beds and chairs, and drugs had been reintroduced, but the focus on diet and health did not change, and water cure continued with state-of-the-art equipment. It transformed to more of a health spa that treated the sick, but no longer accepted "epileptics, and inebriates, among other objectionable cases."[42]

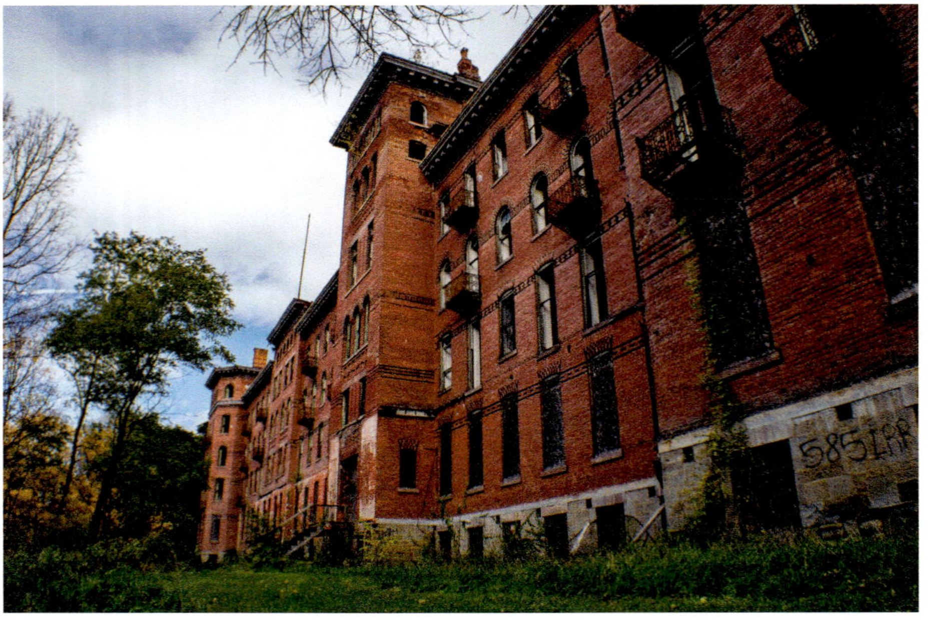

A photo of the red brick façade demonstrates the building's gargantuan size. This six-story edifice is slowly crumbling away with time as wrought-iron balconies oxidize outside their deteriorating arched windows. The orifices to the first two stories, covered in planks of plywood, do not deter trespassers from entering despite its structural integrity nearing collapse. *[Photo by Brian Cray]*

The same treatments still ensued, such as the Moliere-Thermo-Electric Bath, which targeted congestion and inflammation of organs used in cases of gout, rheumatism, catarrh, malaria, and digestive disturbances. It combined heat with electricity, and was practiced for over thirty-five years at the institution.[43] The health resort had four of these bath systems. The Nauheim Bath, which had machines and coils, targeted heart ailments among the Turkish Bath, Russian Bath, Electric Light, Salt and Sulphur Baths, and the administration of shock therapy treatments with the use of statical machines and coils claimed to help with Arterio-Sclerosis, auto-intoxication diseases, enlarged prostates, and high blood pressure.[44] In 1883, a new exercise and massage program was implemented in the health resort, one of the first of its kind in the U.S.A. Influenced by Hartvig Nissen of Norway, they named this section of the spa the Swedish Movement Department.[45] Although the health resort employed many therapies to treat the invalid, it was not only limited to treating the sick. Leisurely activities included swimming down in the pool, and genteel camping was offered to the more hearty patrons, with tents assembled on top of wooden platforms. Some of the gentlemen took up boxing while others participated in the pleasantries of theater.[46]

The Jackson Health Resort was the leading hydrotherapy institute in the world under the Jackson Reign, meeting its demise as the need for water cures dwindled and modern pharmacology replaced it, abandoning operation in 1917.[47] Dr. Jackson died on July 11, 1895, and was buried at Green Mount Cemetery, on a hill, where the rest of the Jacksons lay to rest, looking up at the salubrious sky and scintillating stars, reflecting on their memories of rooftop views from their life's work at the Castle on the Hill.

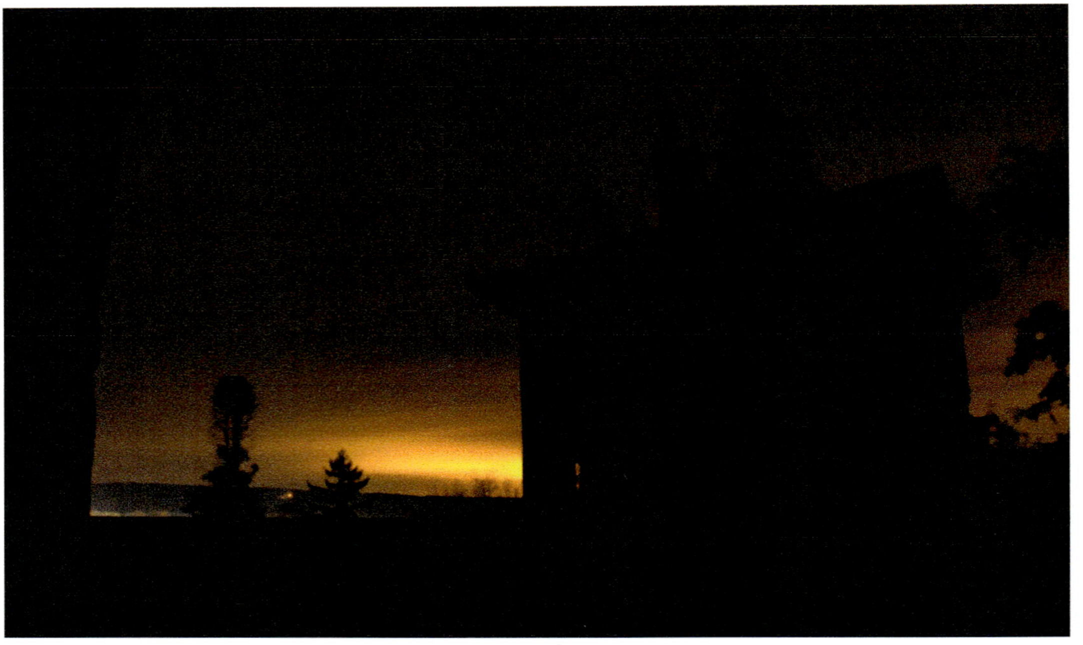

Hours pass and the vibrant blaze fades with the night sky as I look out at Dr. Jackson's office and wonder about the countless nights he must have spent looking out at this very sight. *[Photo by Brian Cray]*

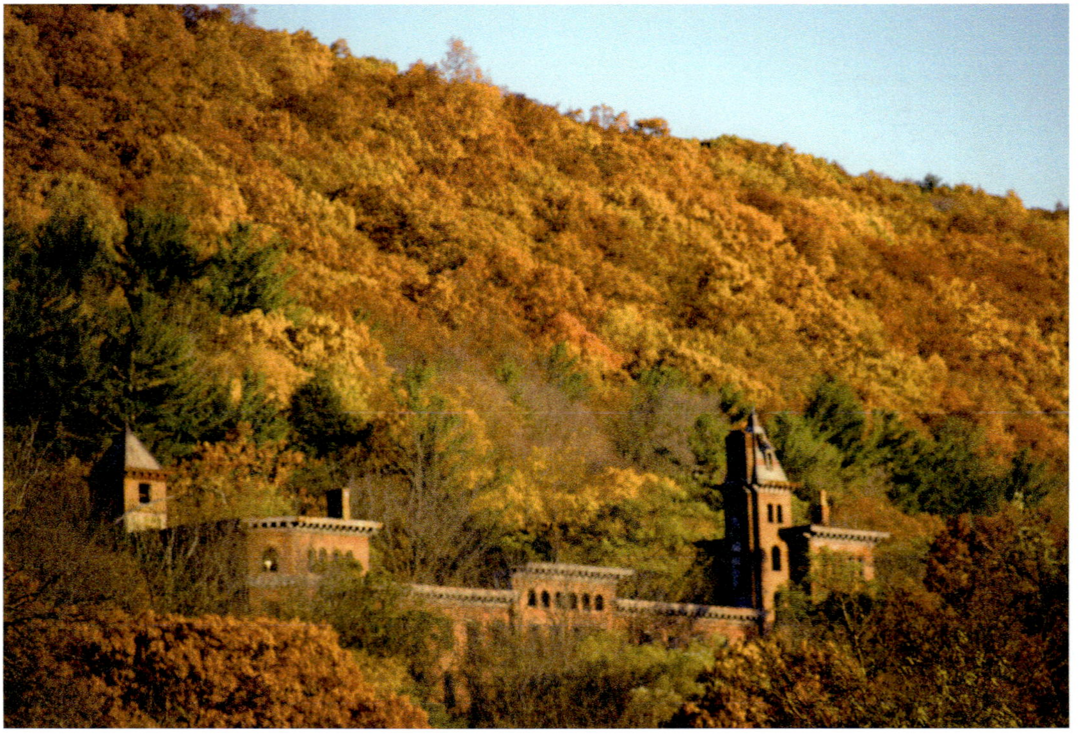

As the cool air strikes the hairs on my neck from Babcock Park, I capture the golden aura of the hillside where the derelict castle withers away with each passing year. *[Photo by Brian Cray]*

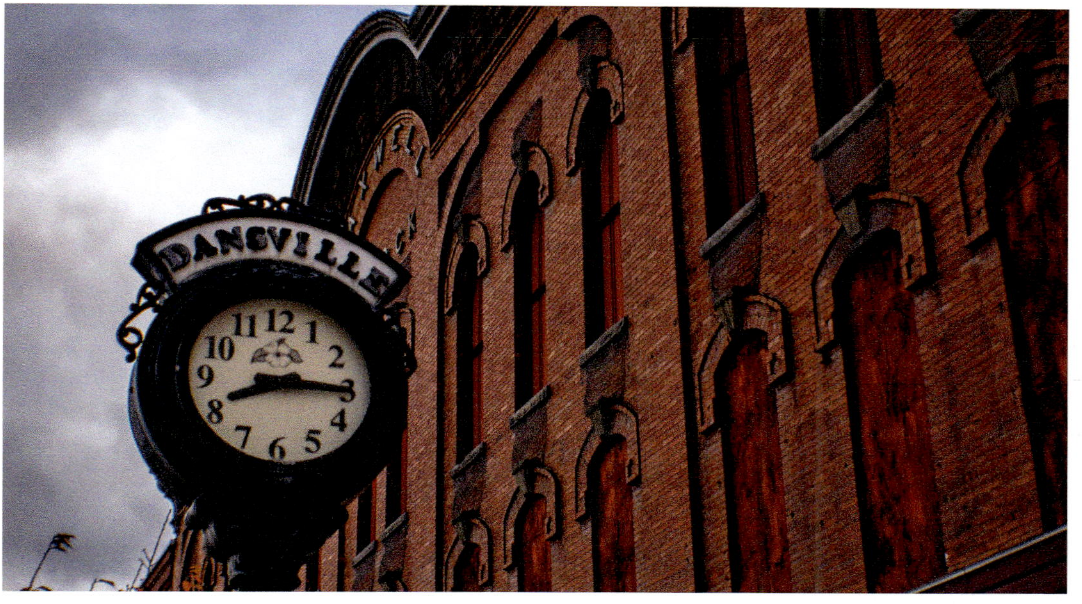

From Main Street in Dansville, the antique clock ticks. The old faded bricks of Maxwell Block make locals ruminate the forgotten memories of its prime era where the Sugar Bowl once resided and the Star Theatre still shines. *[Photo by Brian Cray]*

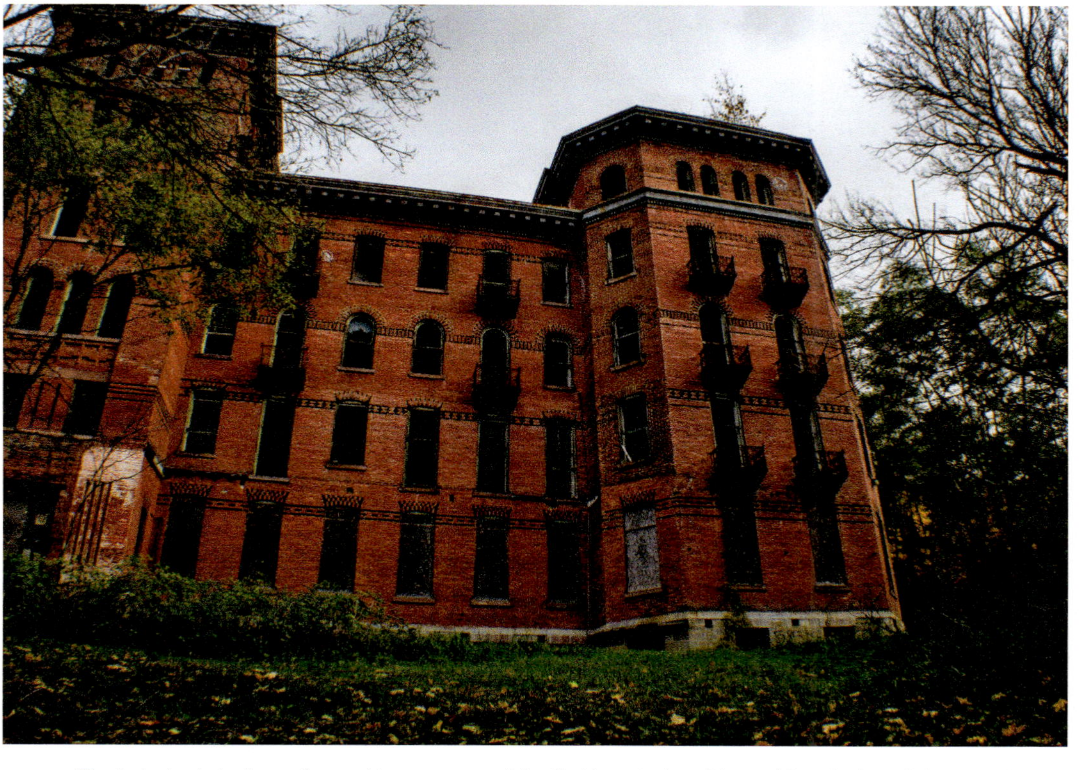

The balustrade to the patio used to wrap around the first two stories of the red façade, but all that remains are boarded windows and oxidized wrought iron balconies of decay. *[Photo by Brian Cray]*

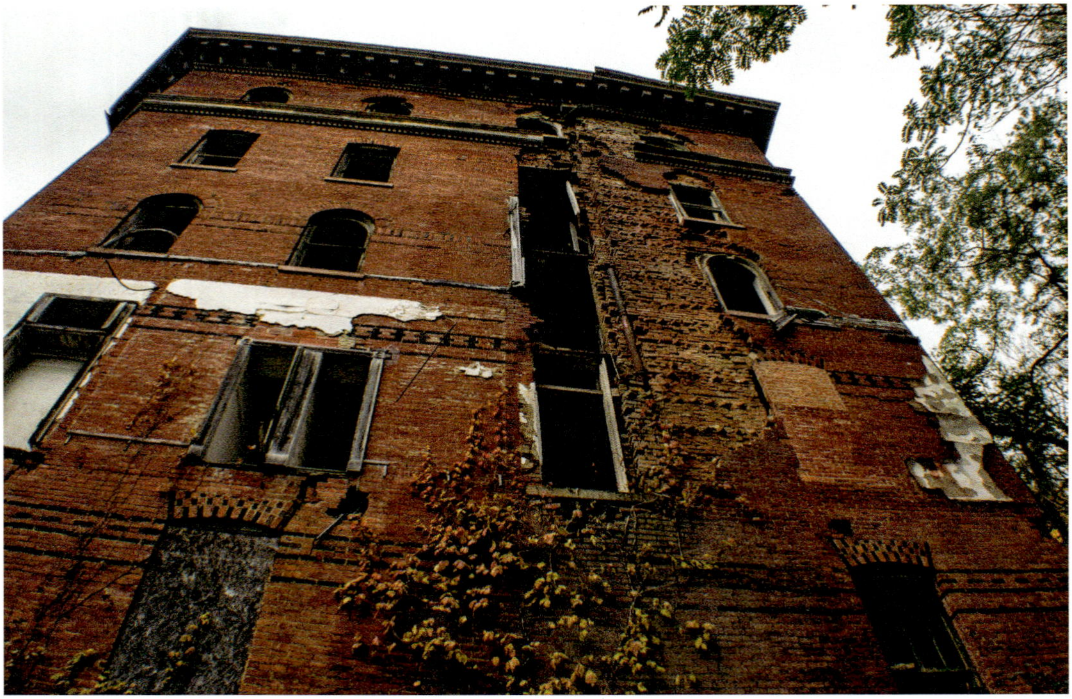

Open doors of brick and broken wood fade to crawling leaves of ivy as she holds back her last breath before collapse. *[Photo by Brian Cray]*

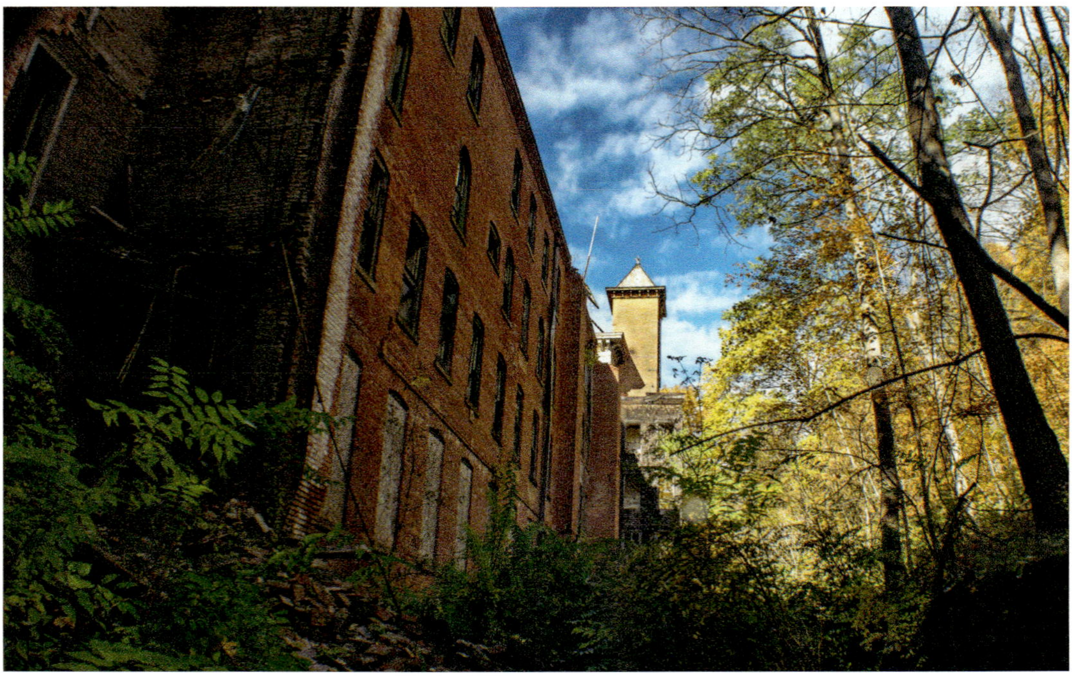

Through deciduous forest and below baby blue sky I see the beautiful decay of a masterpiece slowly slipping away from the community as I wander through her ashes of rubble. *[Photo by Brian Cray]*

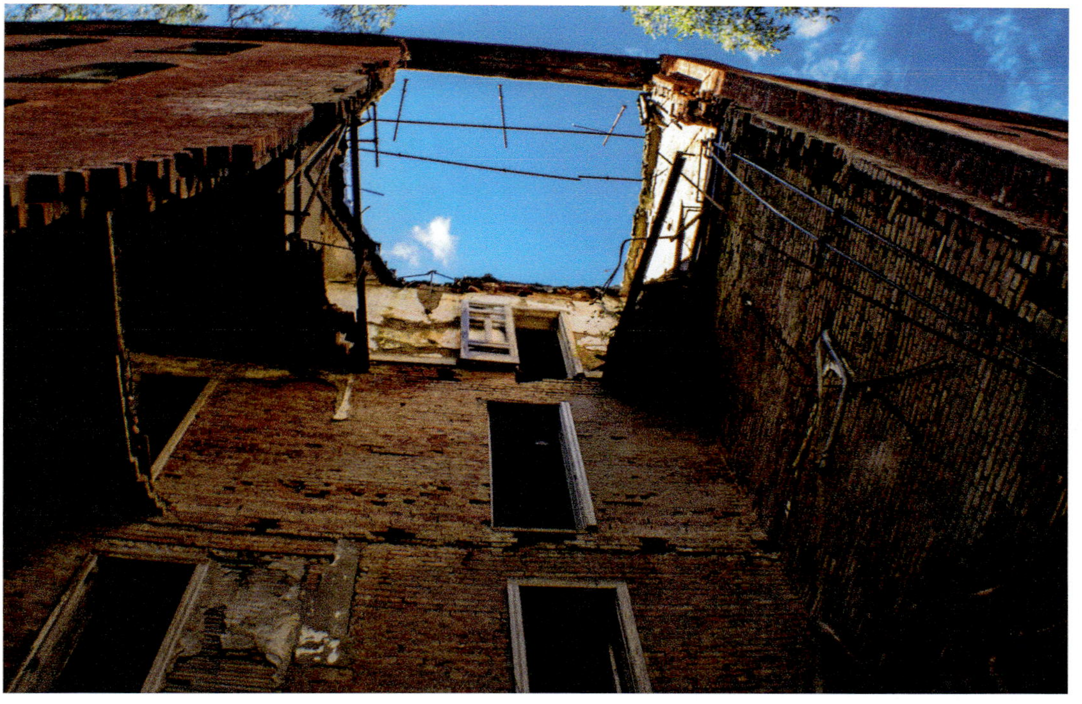

I step closer, looking up at the black pits of loose brick, the ominous doors to nowhere, standing atop the pile of buckled debris from the rooftop, wondering what it was like to dance as a king, overlooking the city. *[Photo by Brian Cray]*

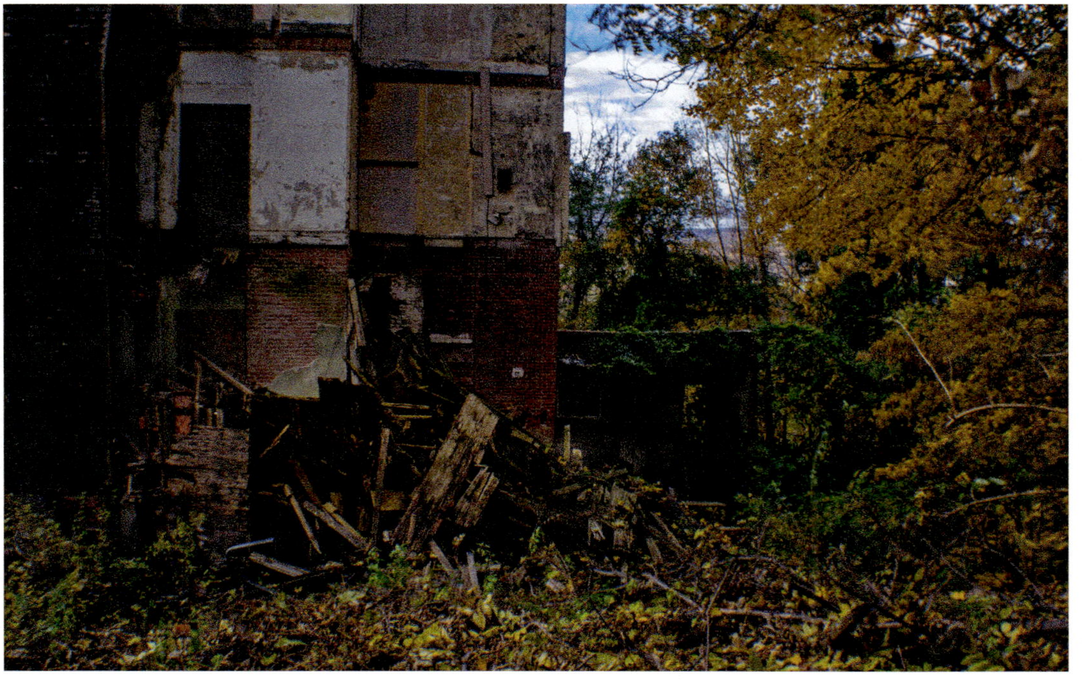

Distorted wood, blackened and splintered, collects mold and mushrooms as the Earth reclaims its forest. *[Photo by Brian Cray]*

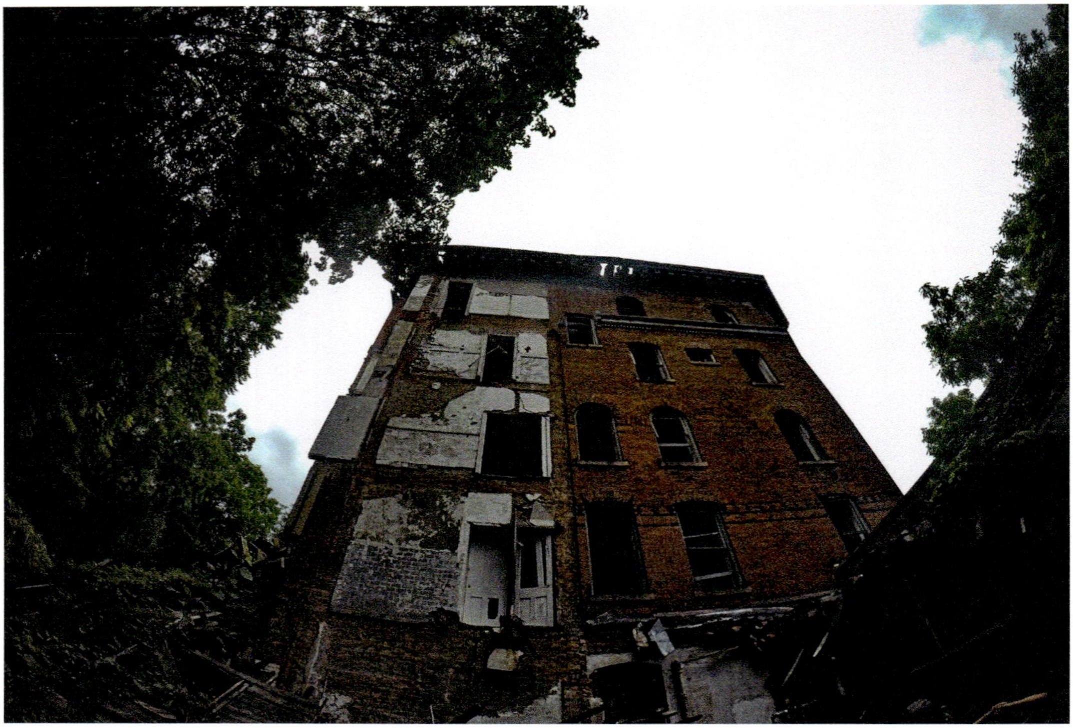

Coniferous forest encroaches on the castle reclaiming bits of earth with the fall of each brick. *[Photo by Brian Cray]*

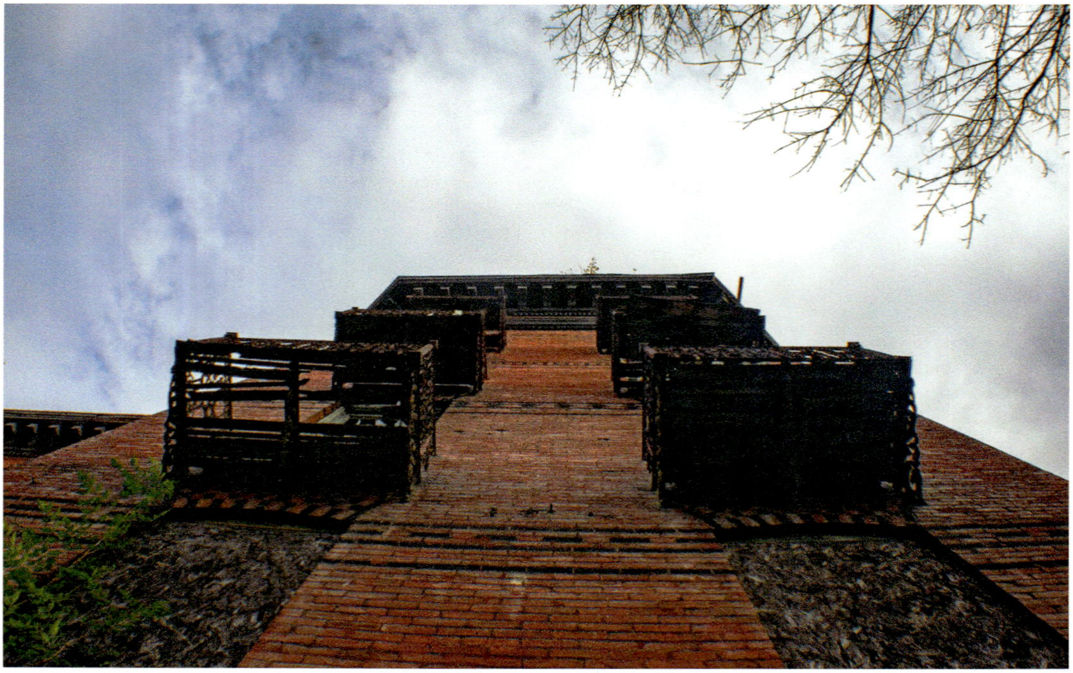

Brittle planks of wood teeter amidst corroded balconies as my eyes crawl up the patterned brick edifice and red fades to clouds. *[Photo by Brian Cray]*

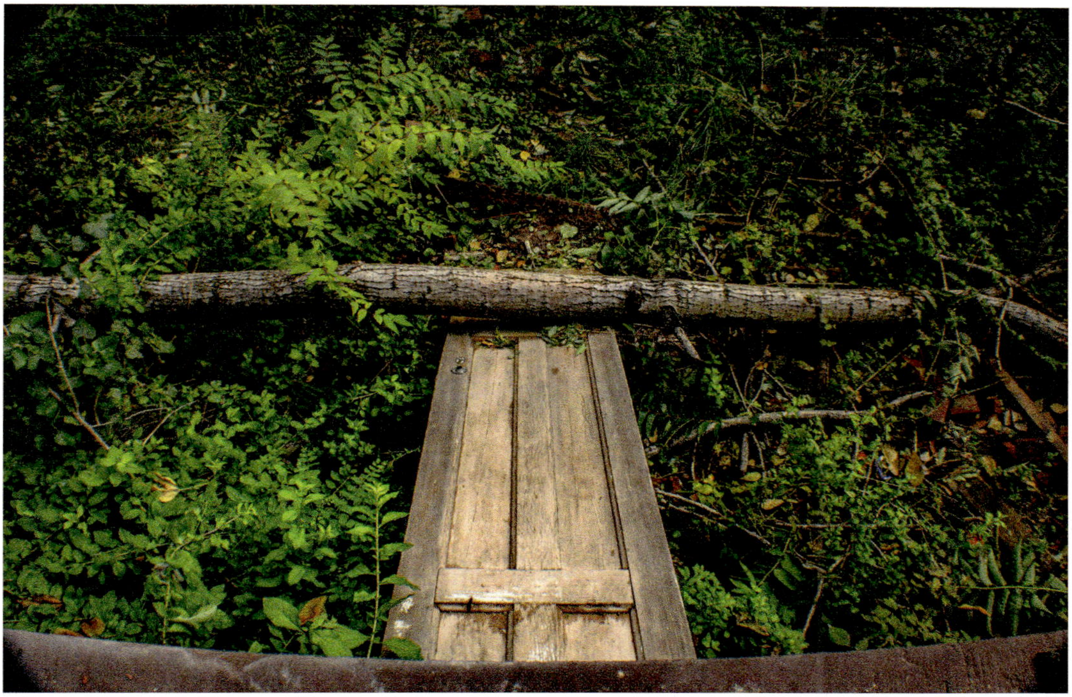

I look down at the perched door covered in dirt and warped from rain. The coarse grains of wood and crevices attract my eyes, but the bright green flowing forest calls my name. *[Photo by Brian Cray]*

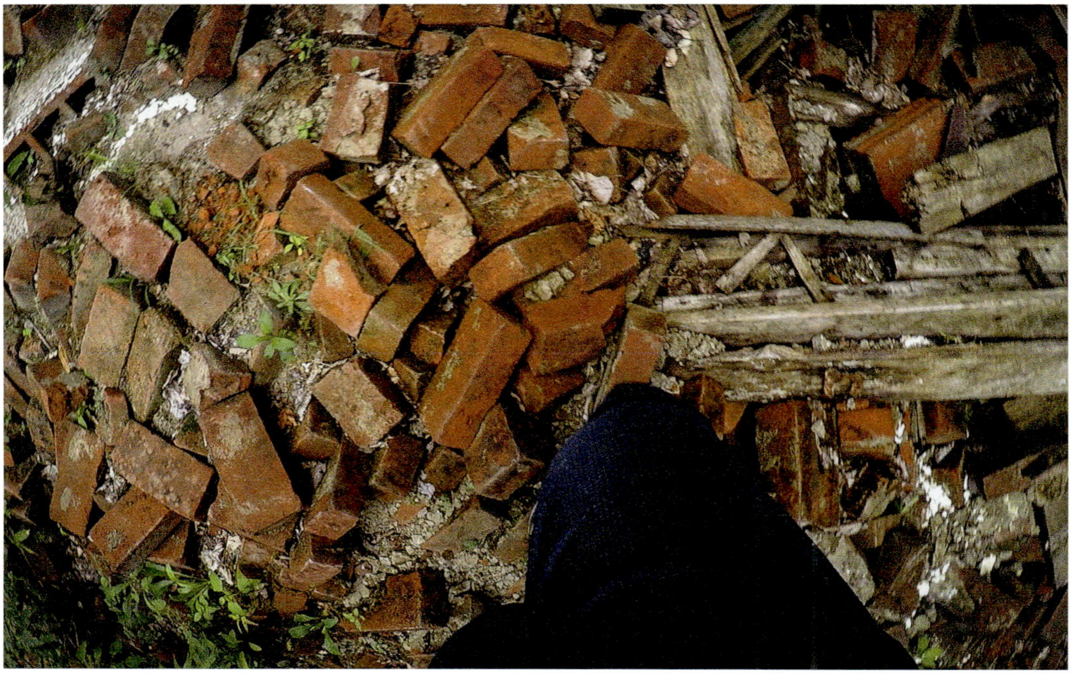

Through the trees, the building screams with her tears piling below in heaps of faded bricks and mangled posts as I look at the façade on the north side of the resort. *[Photo by Brian Cray]*

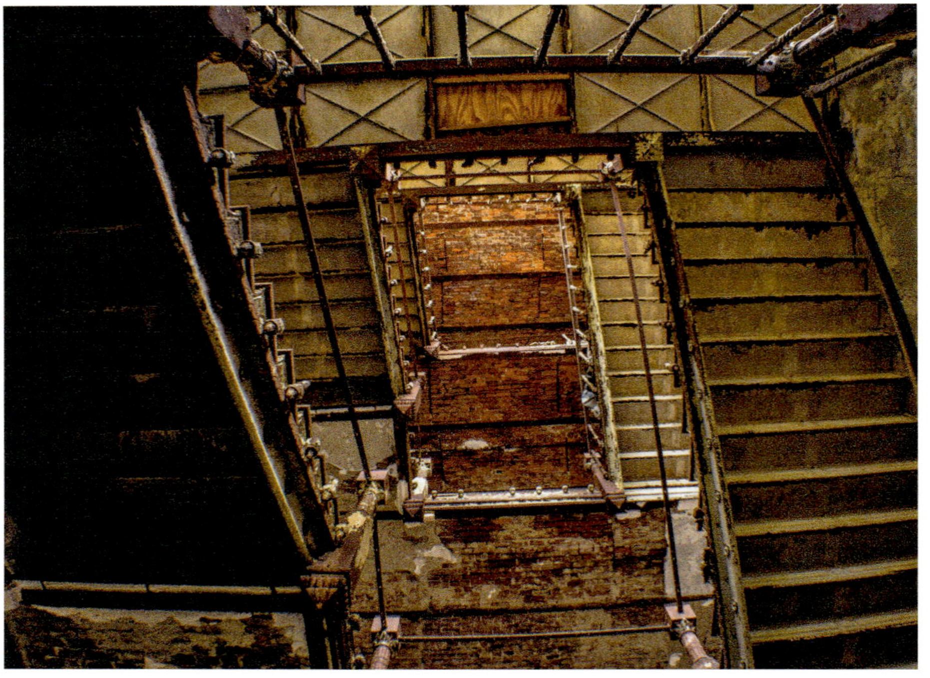

As I leave the clouds of darkness behind reaching the third floor, I peak up through the bleached staircase of tarnished iron and focus on the shades of red immersed in steel and brick. *[Photo by Brian Cray]*

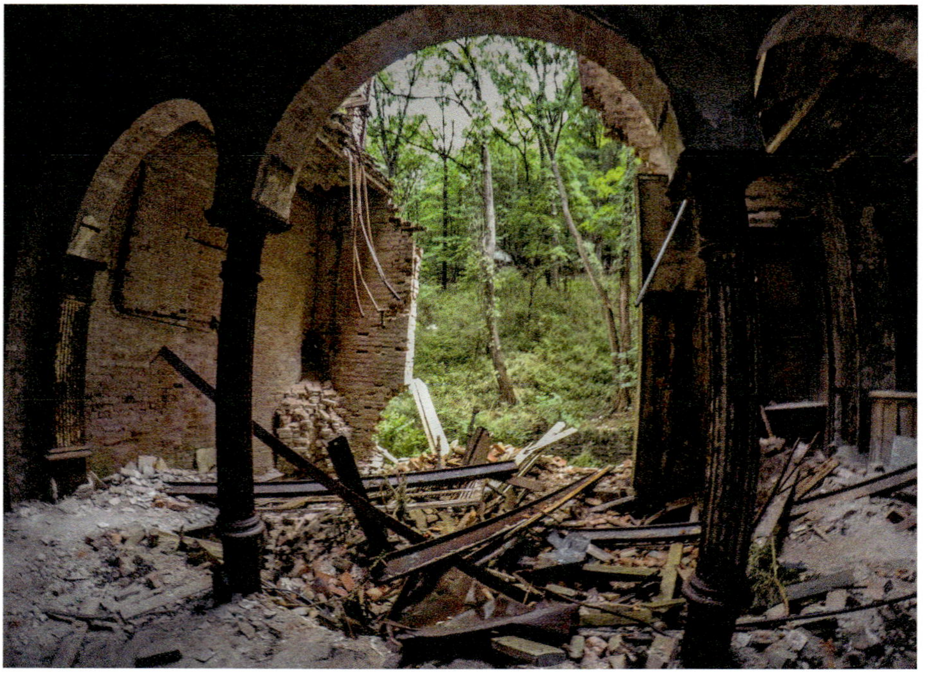

Beyond the arches, steel beams lay awry from the fallen roof. As I look ahead, I try to picture the front desk, but all I see are cracks of crumbling debris, and black voids of barren bricks occupying the ground, stories beneath my shivering toes. *[Photo by Brian Cray]*

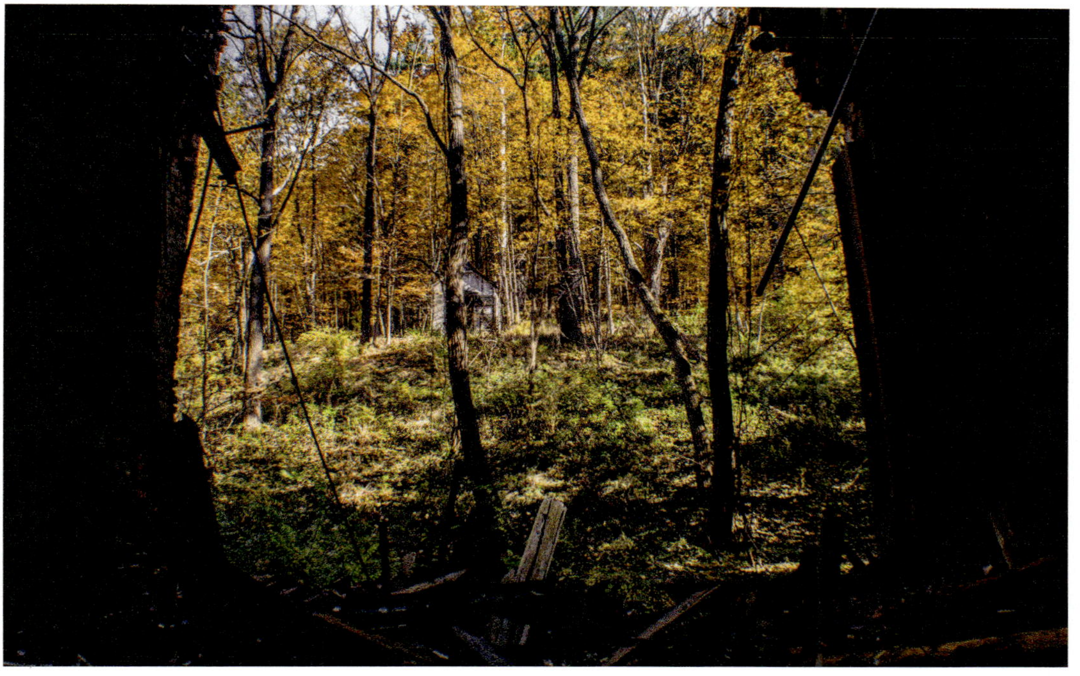

Through the wounded wall of castle I lock onto the chartreuse forest of shimmering leaves and in the distant I spot an old, intact, shed. *[Photo by Brian Cray]*

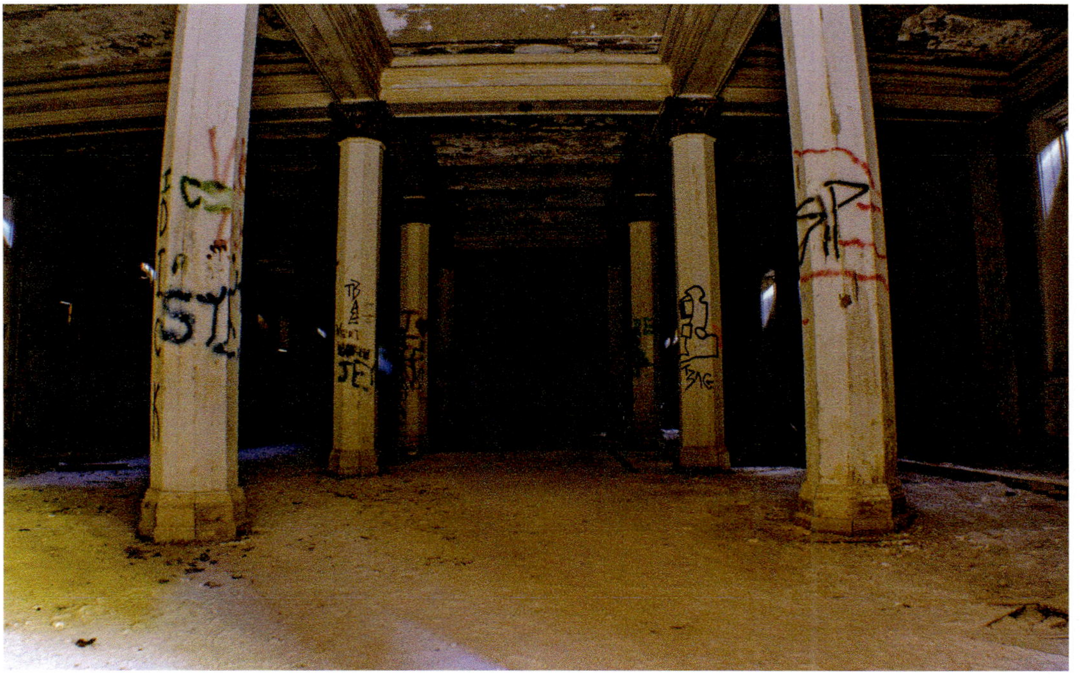

Corinthian columns march off into the abyss while clouds of dust suffocate my lungs as I step deeper into oblivion. At one time the hardwood floors, ivory walls and ornate Ancient Greek columns gave life to the dining room, but now they wither away in shadows of decay. *[Photo by Brian Cray]*

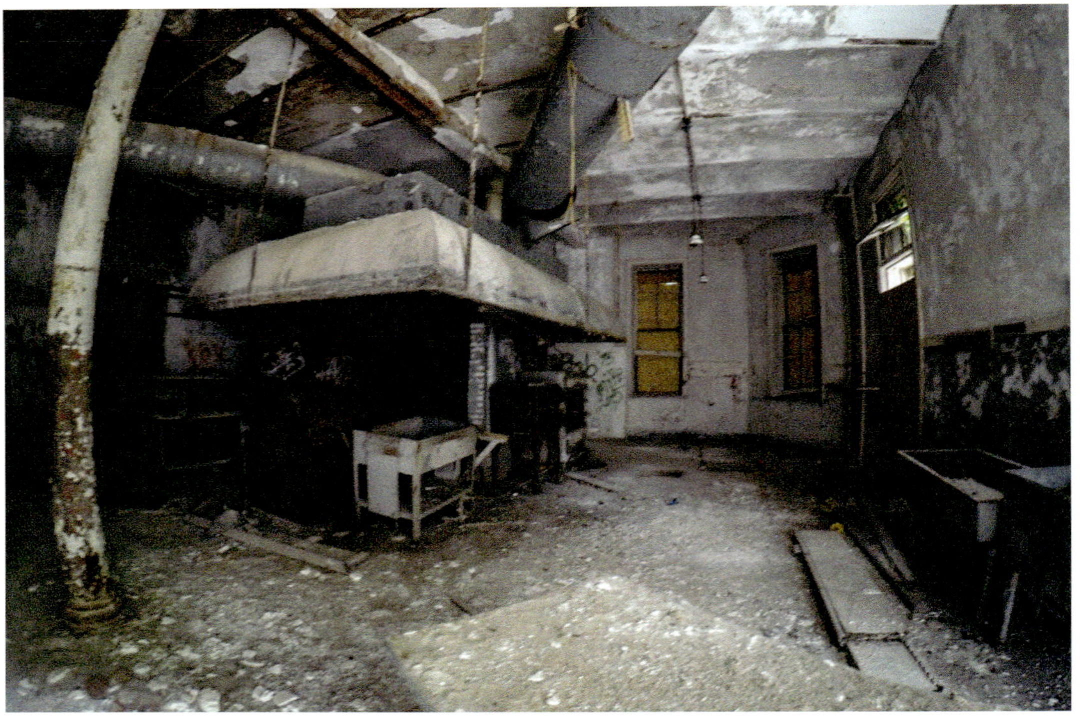

This is what I would presume to be the kitchen to the Jackson Sanatorium, with multiple sinks and a ventilation system for the stoves. *[Photo by Brian Cray]*

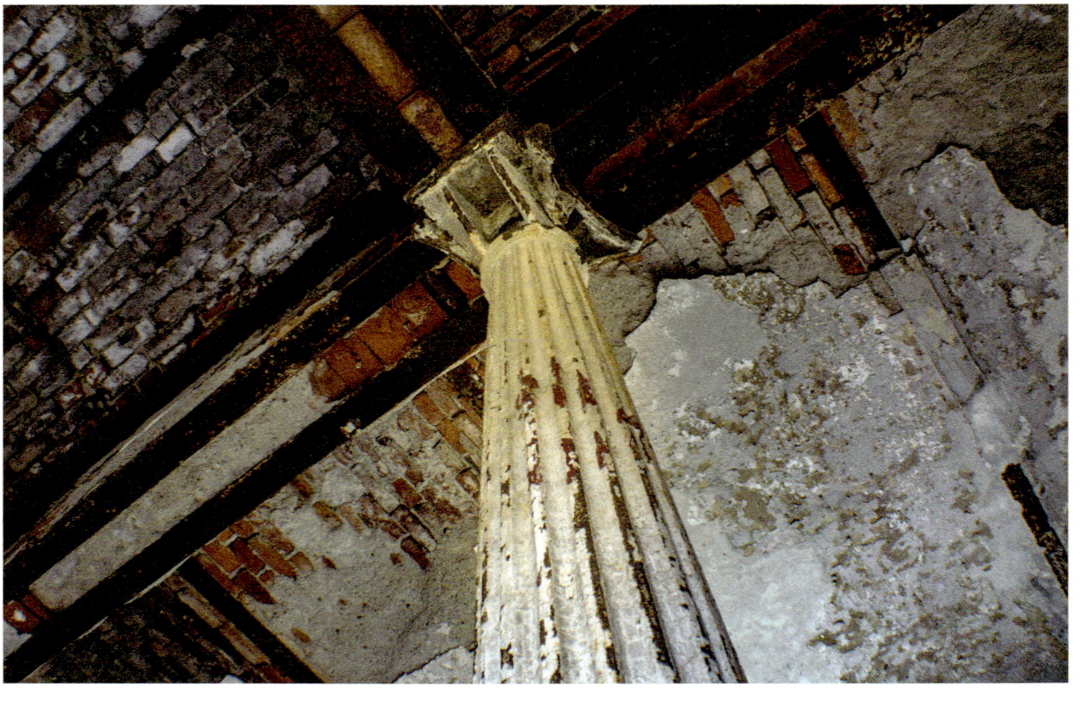

Corinthian columns flake away ivory as the prowess of the castle stands in brick and steel. *[Photo by Brian Cray]*

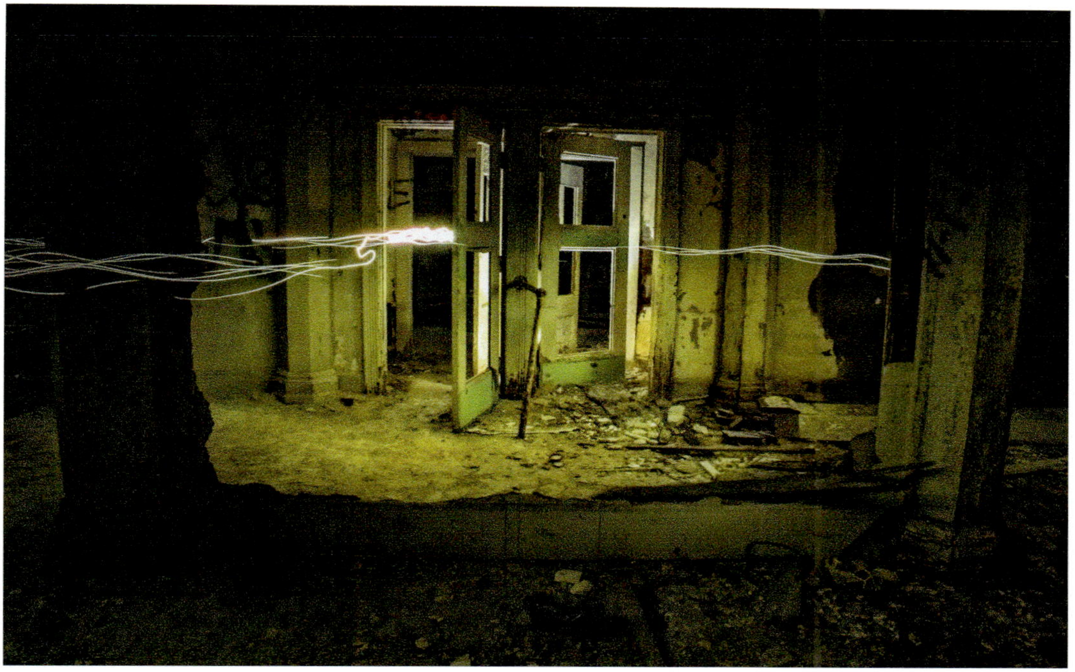

All lights lead directly to the kitchen through paneless doors and broken walls where everything fades to black. *[Photo by Brian Cray]*

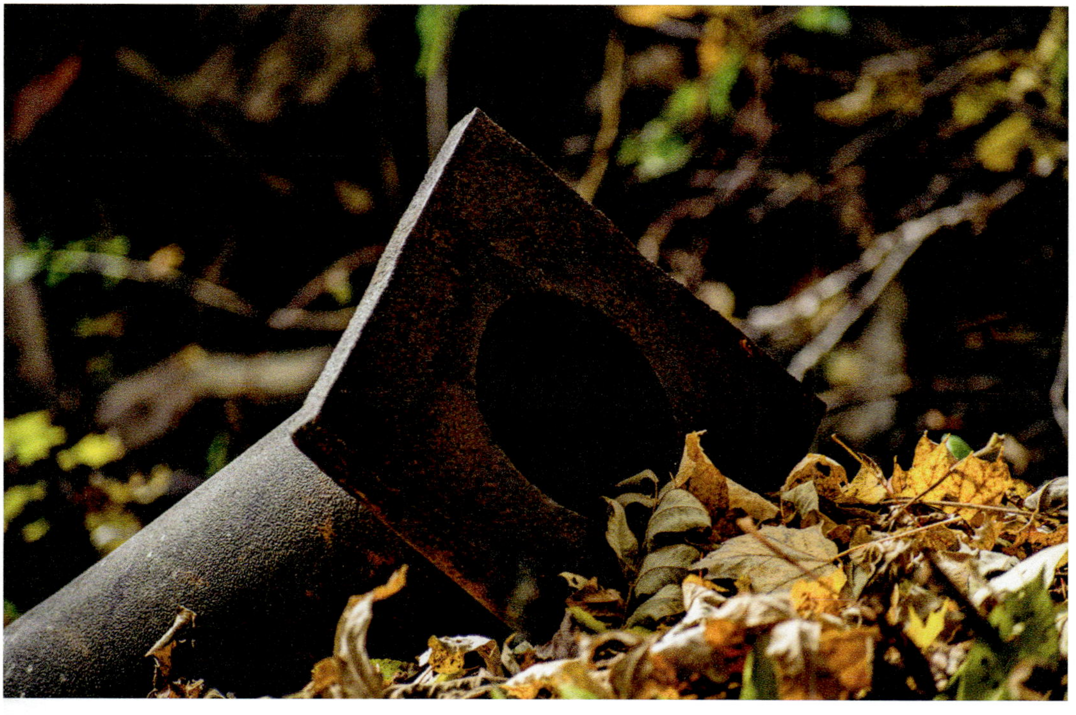

An iron column flaked in rust decays on the hillside amongst the forest. *[Photo by Brian Cray]*

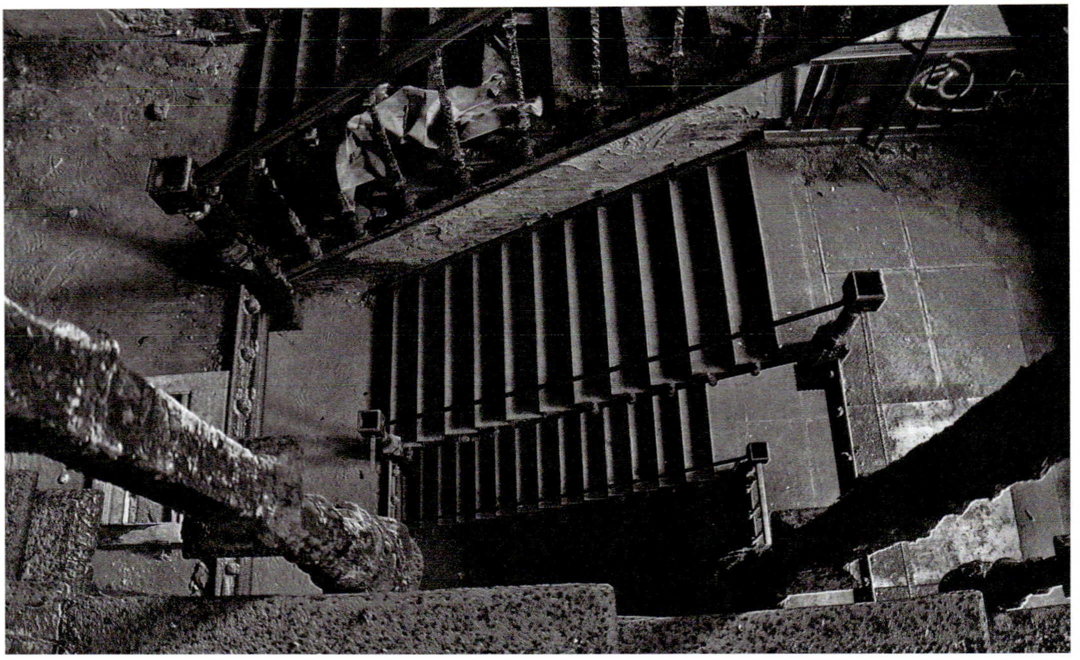

Macfadden opened his first health resort outside of Manhattan and called it Macfadden Health Home. He mocked the medical world by issuing a statement saying he would cure the sick through natural means and free-of-charge. (Adams, 2010) *[Photo by Brian Cray]*

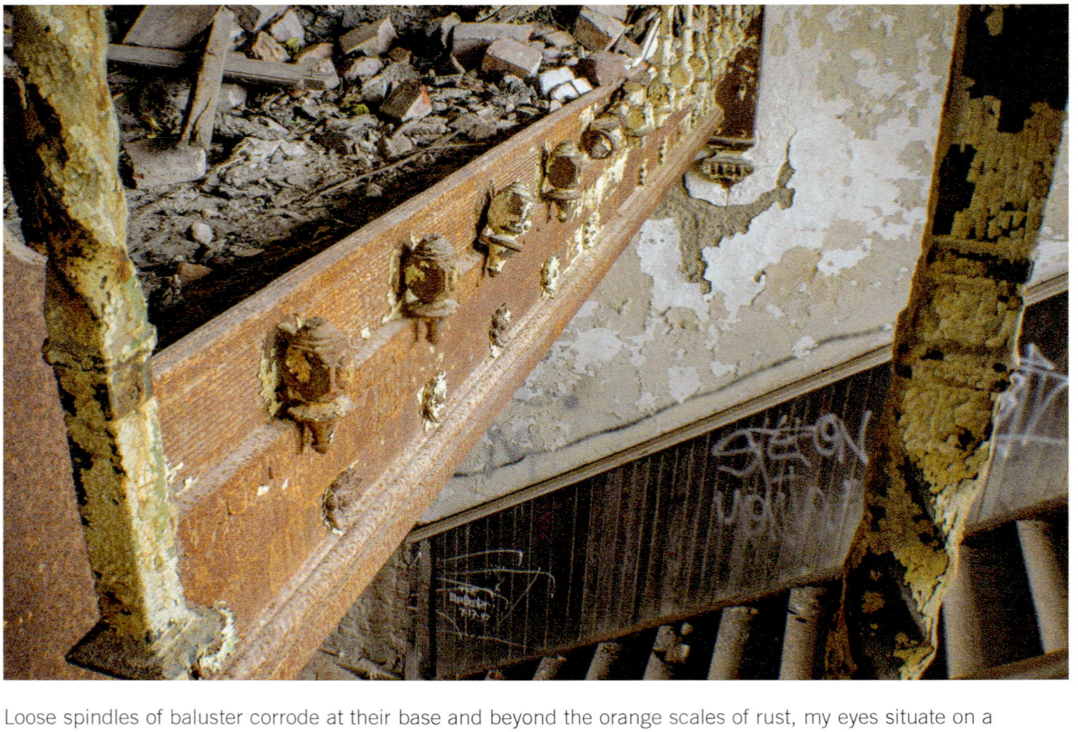

Loose spindles of baluster corrode at their base and beyond the orange scales of rust, my eyes situate on a mound of rubble and loose debris from the rooftop. *[Photo by Brian Cray]*

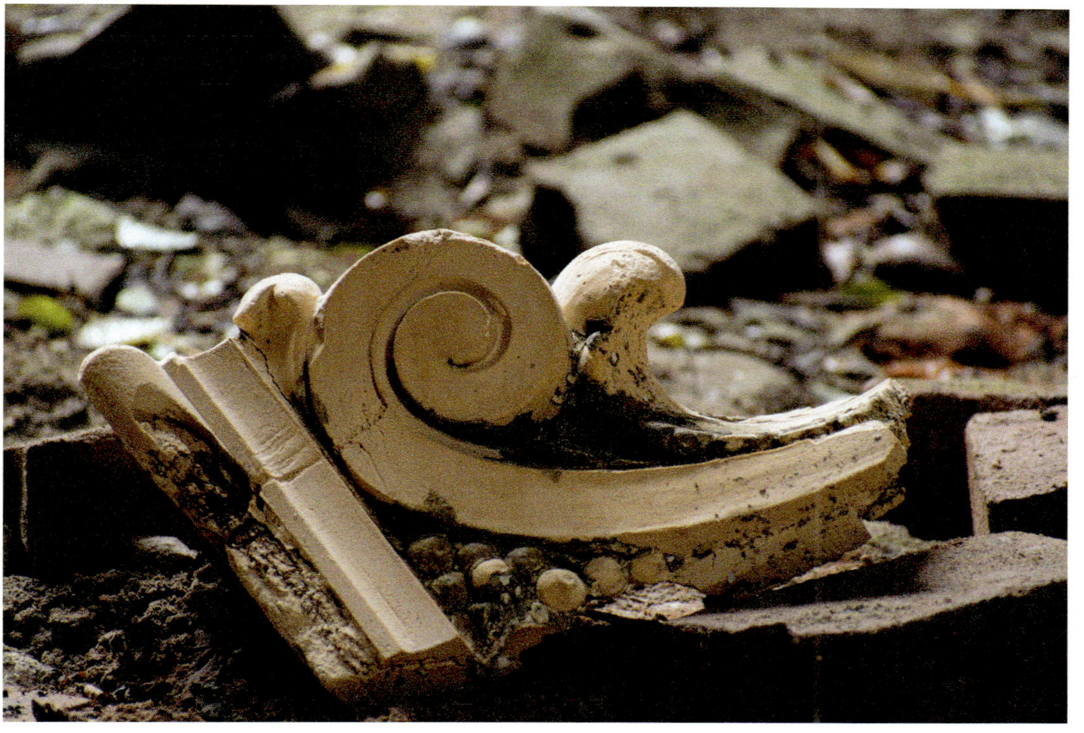

Bits of loose brick, smidgeons of dust, and dirt and splinters of wood circle the broken pink crown of a Corinthian column. I shut my eyes and imagine the intricate grooves and details decorating the halls as patrons wander around through the castle and I smile. *[Photo by Brian Cray]*

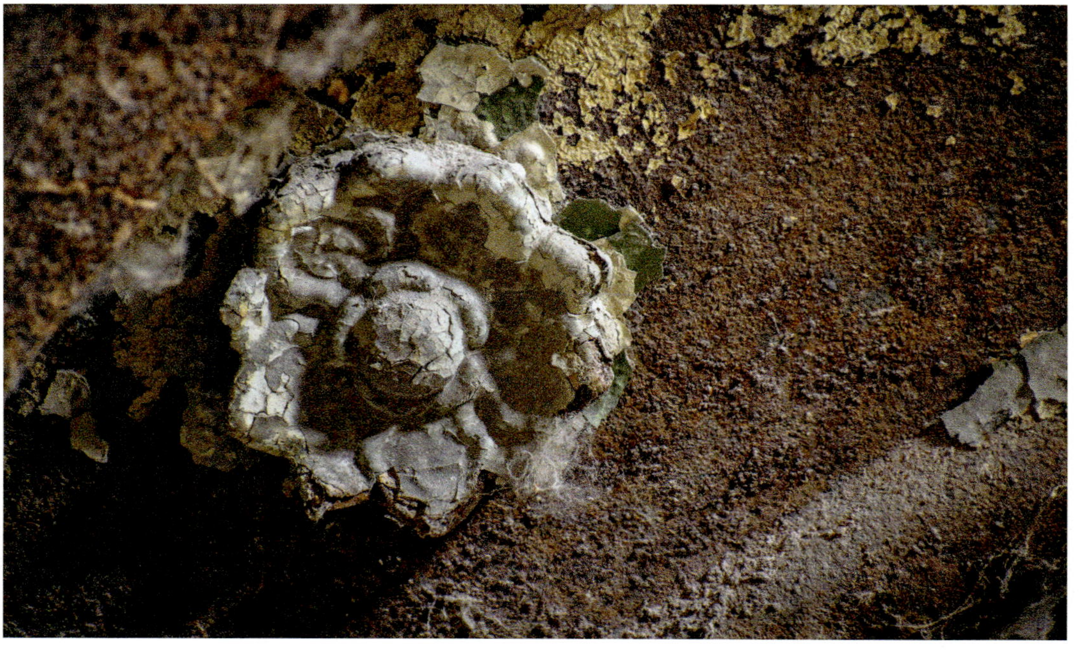

Fissures of paint chip away at the rosettes marching up the iron molding of the staircase. *[Photo by Brian Cray]*

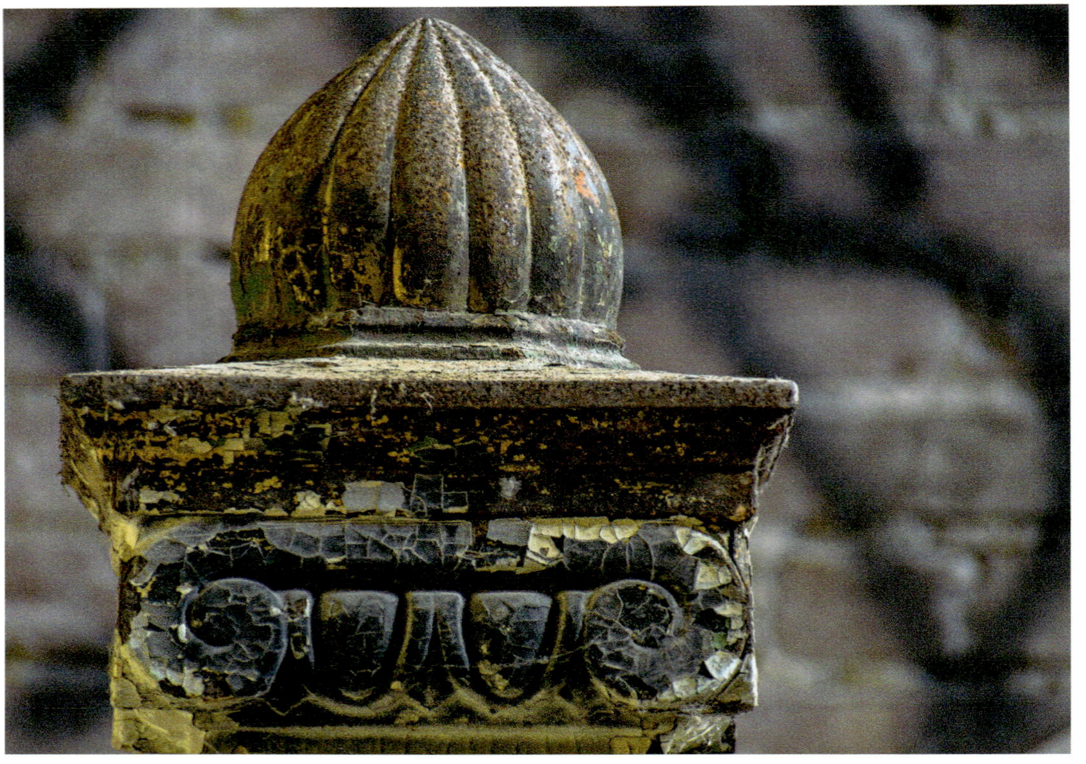

Beneath the cracks and exposed paint, splotches of rust corrode away at the newel post to an otherwise beautiful balustrade. *[Photo by Brian Cray]*

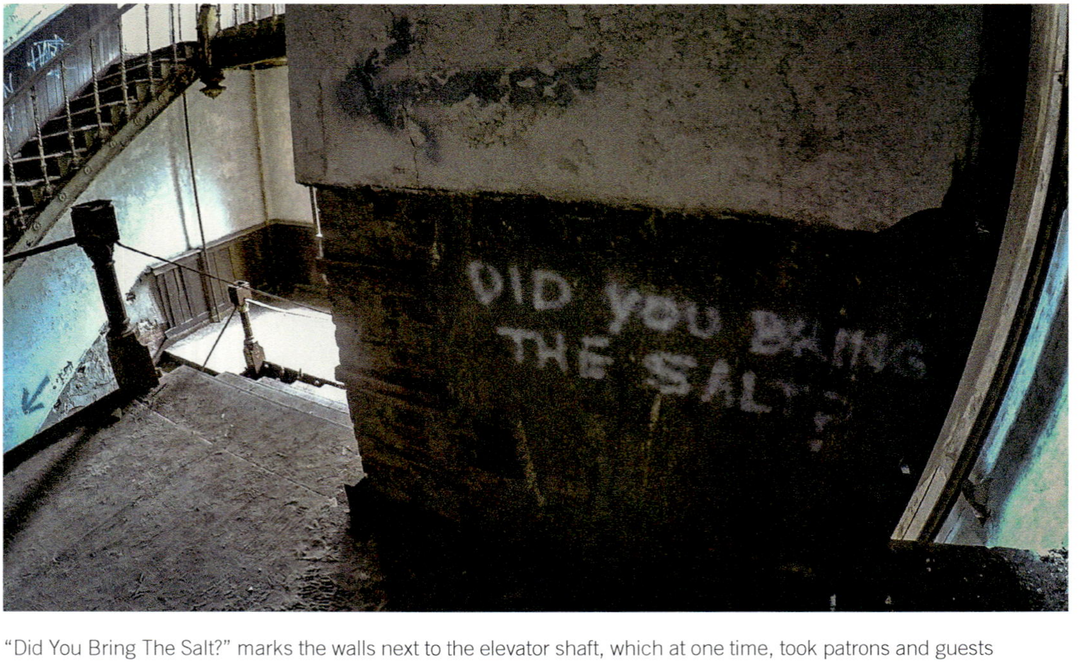

"Did You Bring The Salt?" marks the walls next to the elevator shaft, which at one time, took patrons and guests to the rooftop to dance among the gardens or sunbathe in the towers. *[Photo by Brian Cray]*

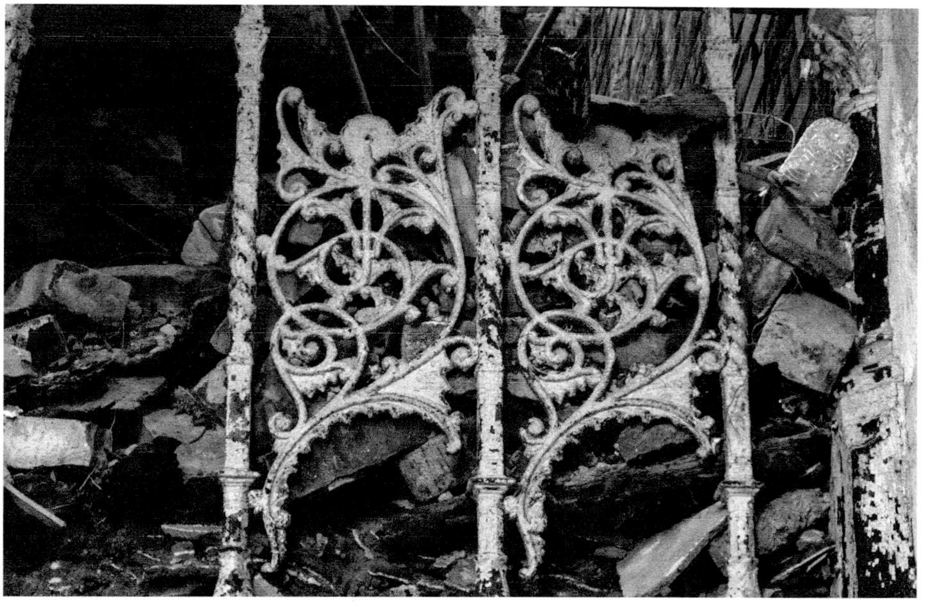

The only two balusters that have not completely perished to broken spindles of time. Macfadden would go on to open his second health home a year later in 1902 along Lake Ronkonkoma for profit, but within a short seven-month timeframe, he closed its doors due to unreliable help and thievery (Adams, 2010). *[Photo by Brian Cray]*

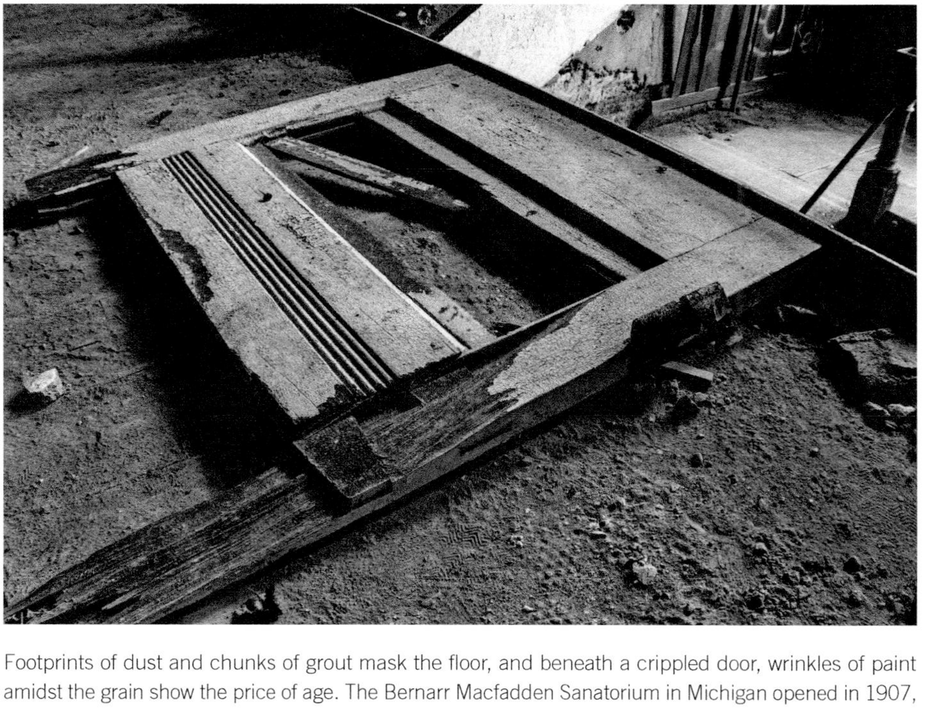

Footprints of dust and chunks of grout mask the floor, and beneath a crippled door, wrinkles of paint amidst the grain show the price of age. The Bernarr Macfadden Sanatorium in Michigan opened in 1907, competing with Battle Creek Sanitarium. This gargantuan building featured Russian and Turkish baths, swimming pools, a gymnasium among other amenities geared towards promoting "Physcultopathy" methods, which aimed for a new science of healing. (Adams, 2010) *[Photo by Brian Cray]*

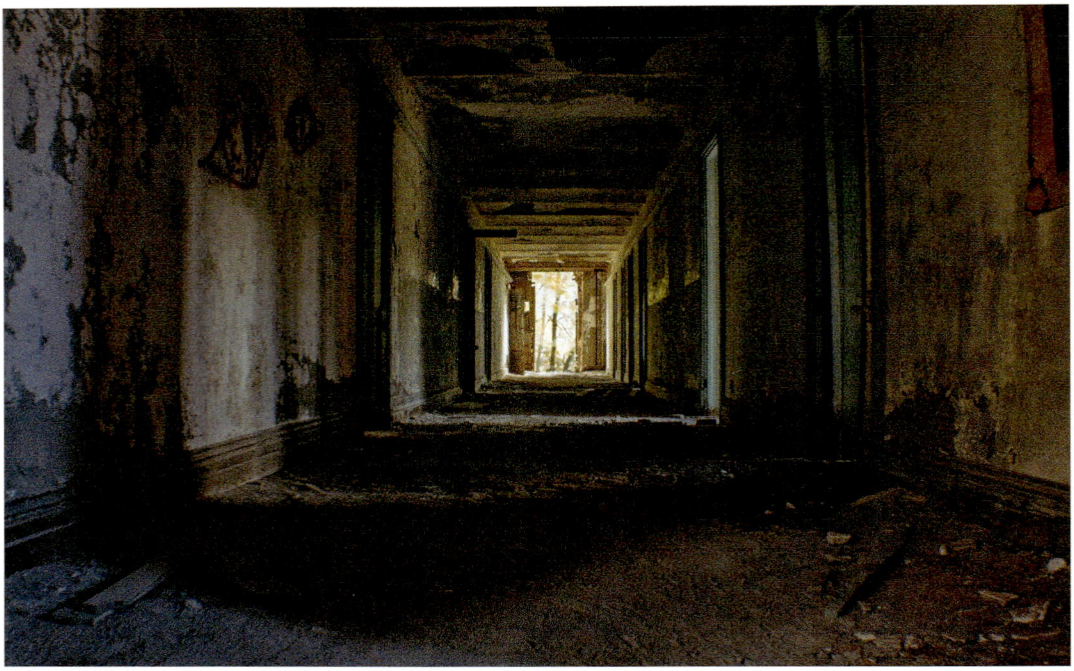

The empty halls of tortured walls, swathed in shadows of crumbling age, wait in pain for her last brick to fall as I gaze to the forest beyond. *[Photo by Brian Cray]*

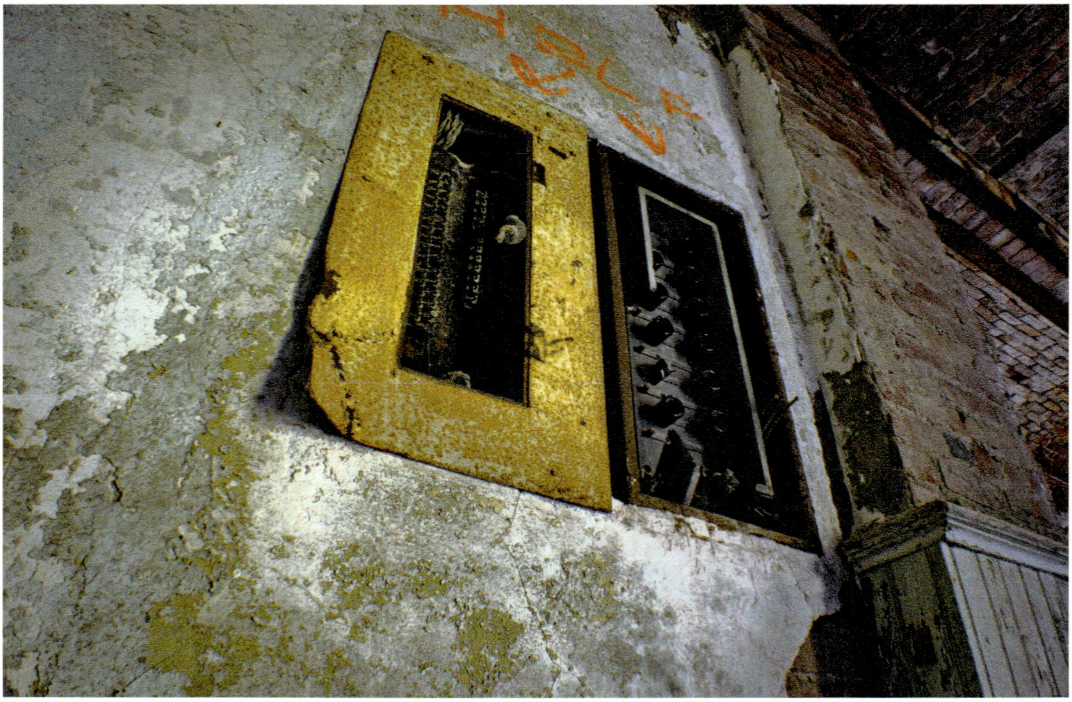

Dappled dots mark the coarse metal like Braille as my fingers softly trail the frame of the breaker. *[Photo by Brian Cray]*

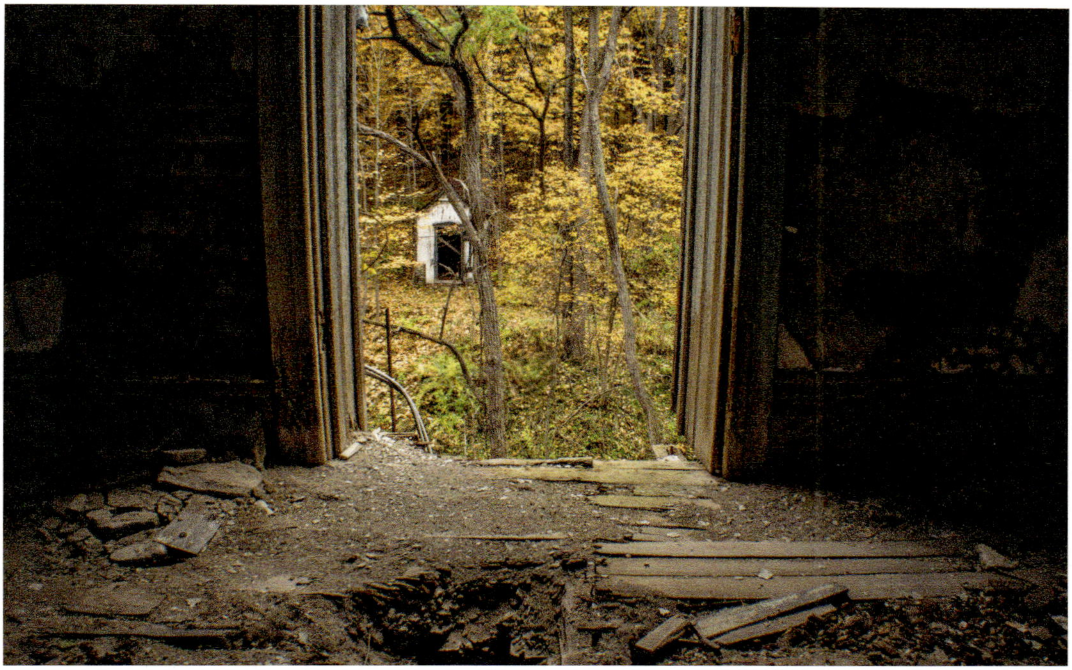

As my eyes wander past the mangled floorboards and bits of plaster, they widen at the orifice of missing bricks chiseled out of the floor like Jenga pieces. The shed looms off in the distance and I falter back to sturdy ground in fear. *[Photo by Brian Cray]*

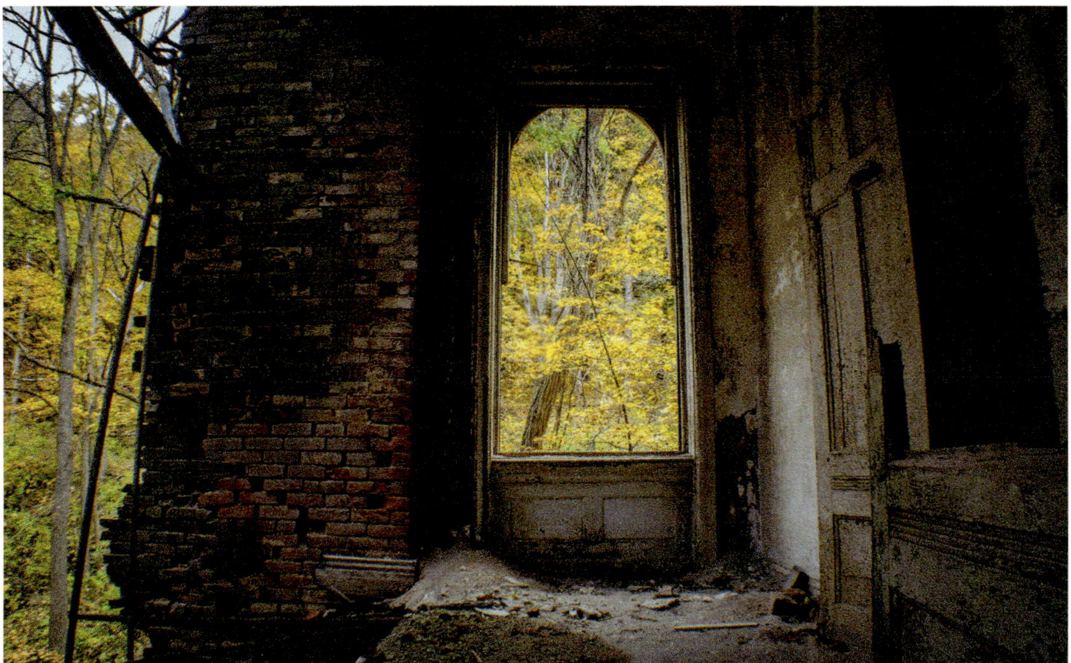

Pits of faded, crumbling bricks, mounds of rubble and dust and bent pipes cannot distract me from the canvas of vibrant yellows flourishing beyond her distressed walls. *[Photo by Brian Cray]*

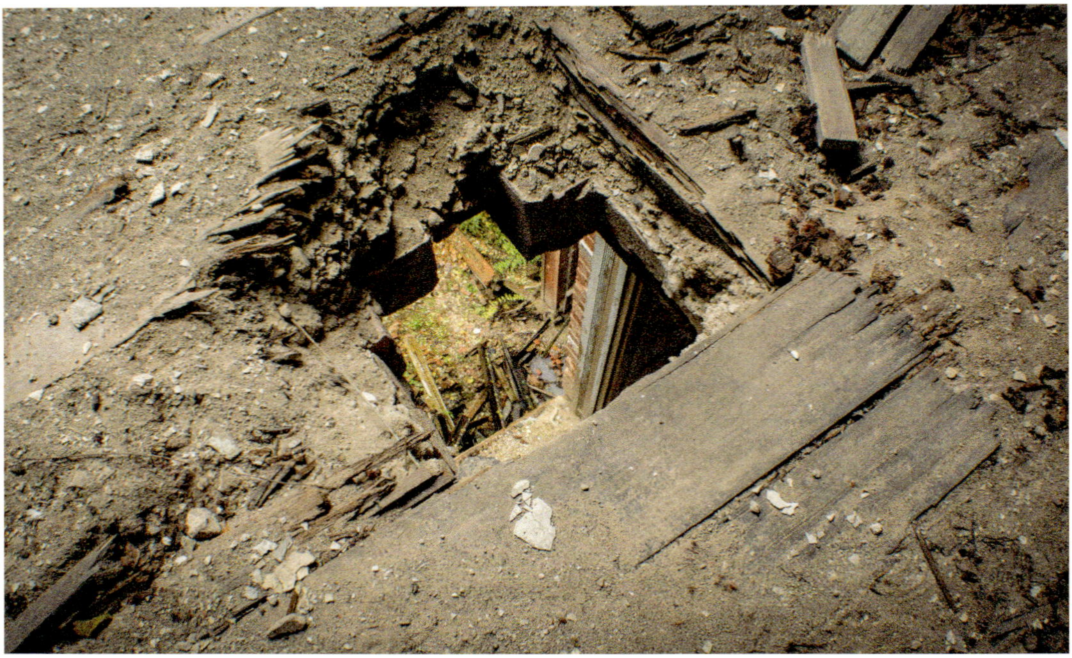

Watch your step and don't look down! The first floor is closer than she looks! *[Photo by Brian Cray]*

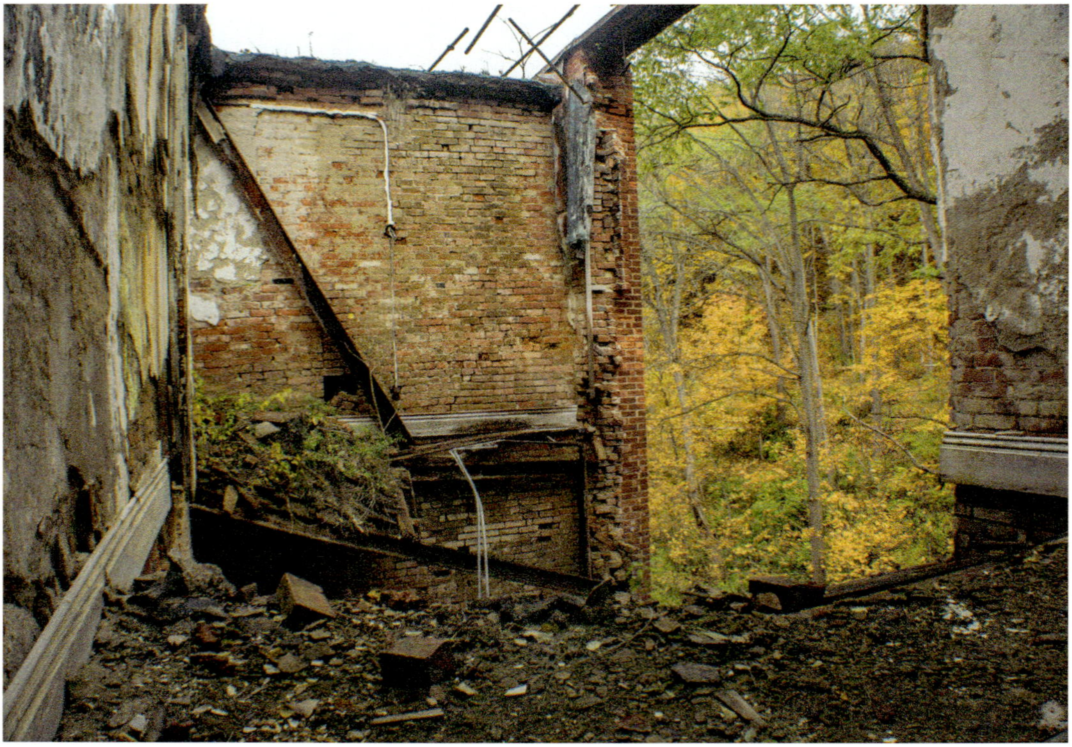

Here I stand, so close, but yet so far from my long journey to the roof. Her bowed steel beams flounder between loose bricks as I pitter back inside. *[Photo by Brian Cray]*

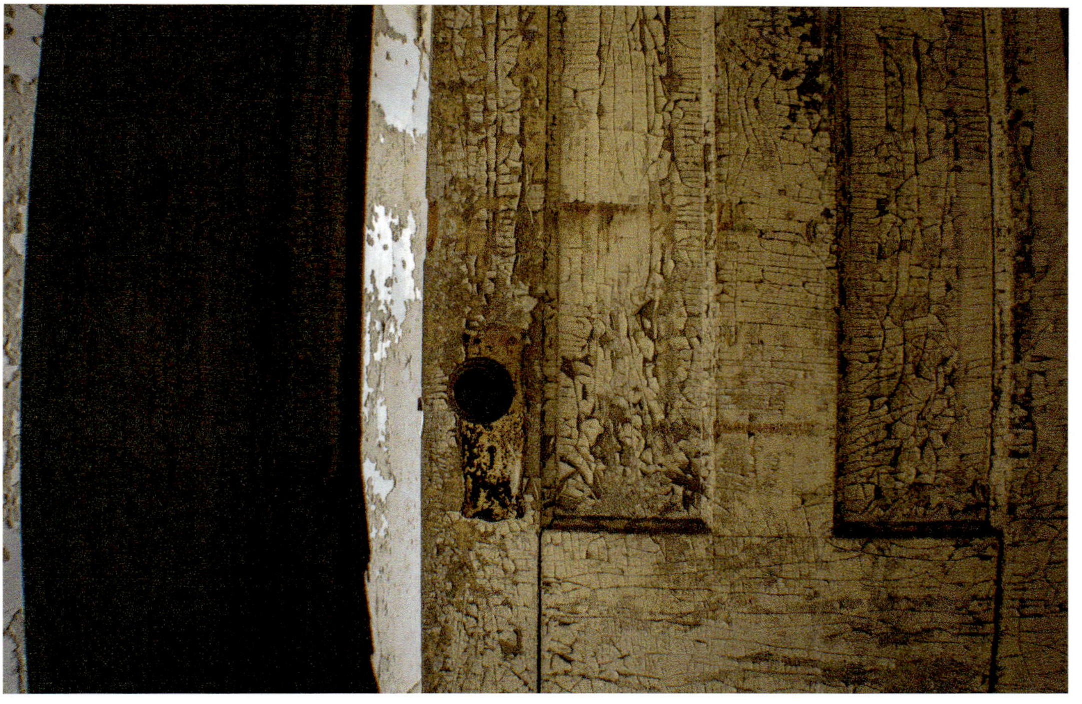

Dull paint curls back along the crackled grain as I reach for the rusty handle stained with age. *[Photo by Brian Cray]*

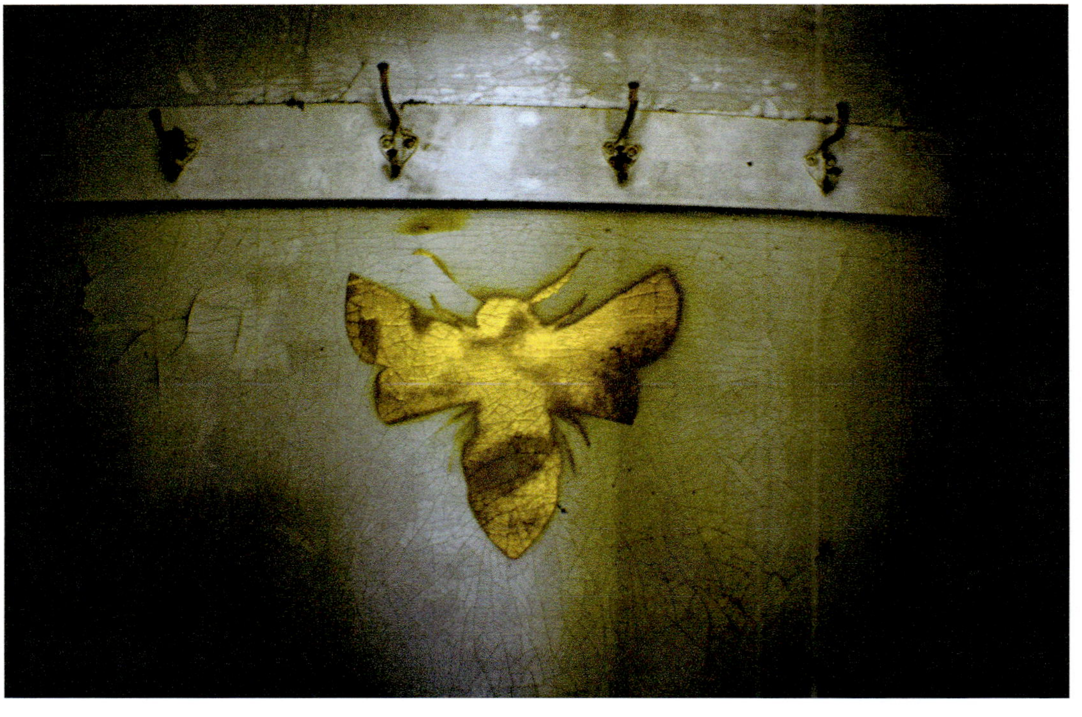

Through all the heinous scribbling tarnishing her walls, I cast my eyes upon a golden butterfly. For a moment, it triggered splendor of what once was a masterpiece of architecture. *[Photo by Brian Cray]*

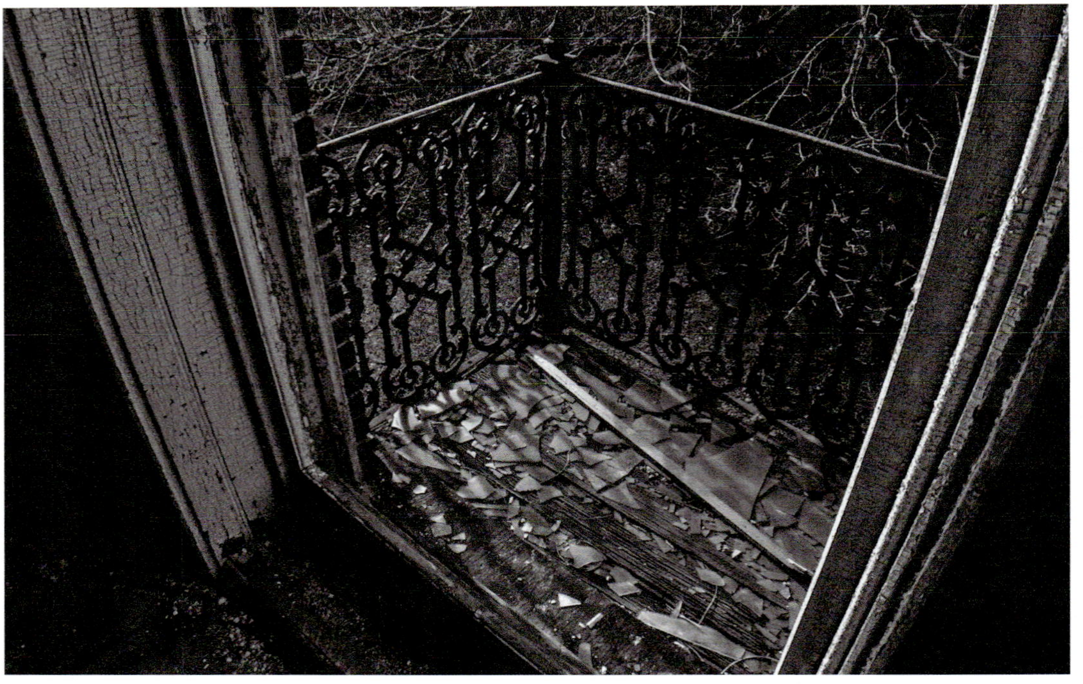

Shattered glass and twisted wood blanket the brittle balcony and all I can focus on are the eerie shadows cast from the falling sun. The Bernarr Macfadden Sanatorium in Michigan only lasted two years due to discrepancies in the purchase agreement so he moved yet again. (Adams, 2010) *[Photo by Brian Cray]*

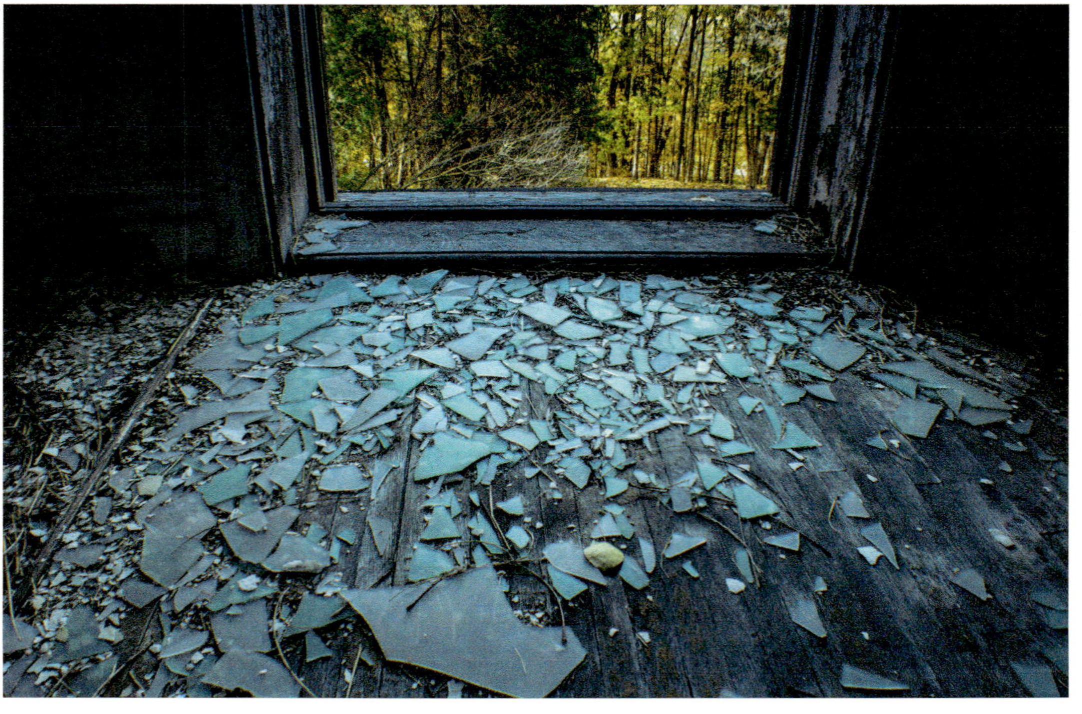

Shattered bits of blue. Pierce my eyes like the ocean. Glass shrieks under foot. *[Photo by Brian Cray]*

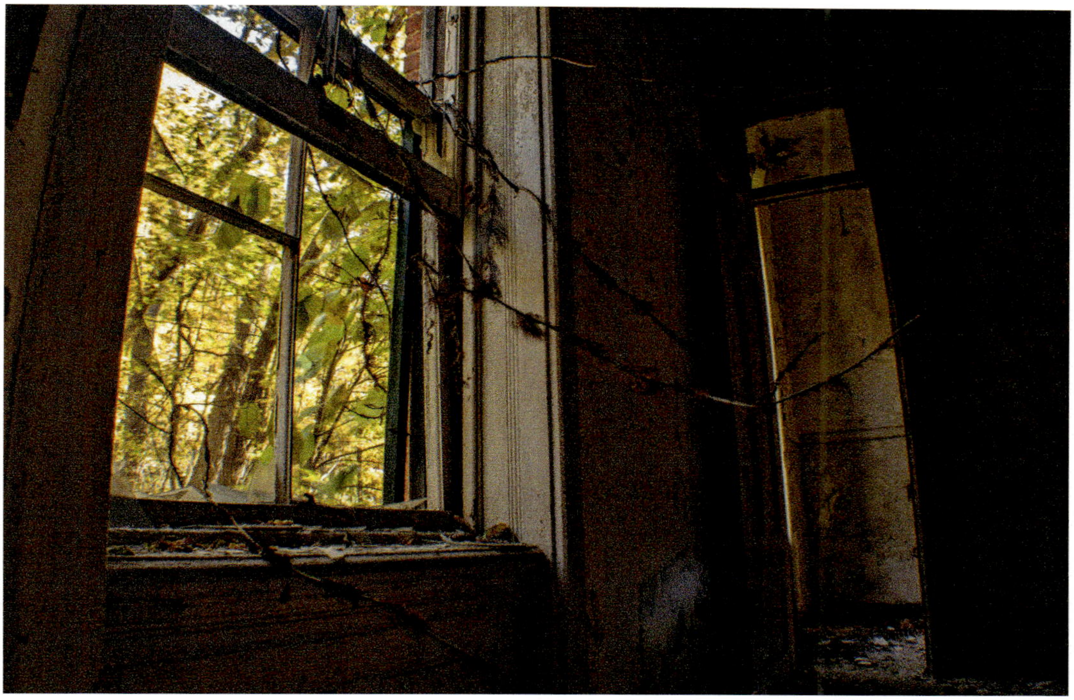

Dead ivy binds around the window frame like twisted limbs. *[Photo by Brian Cray]*

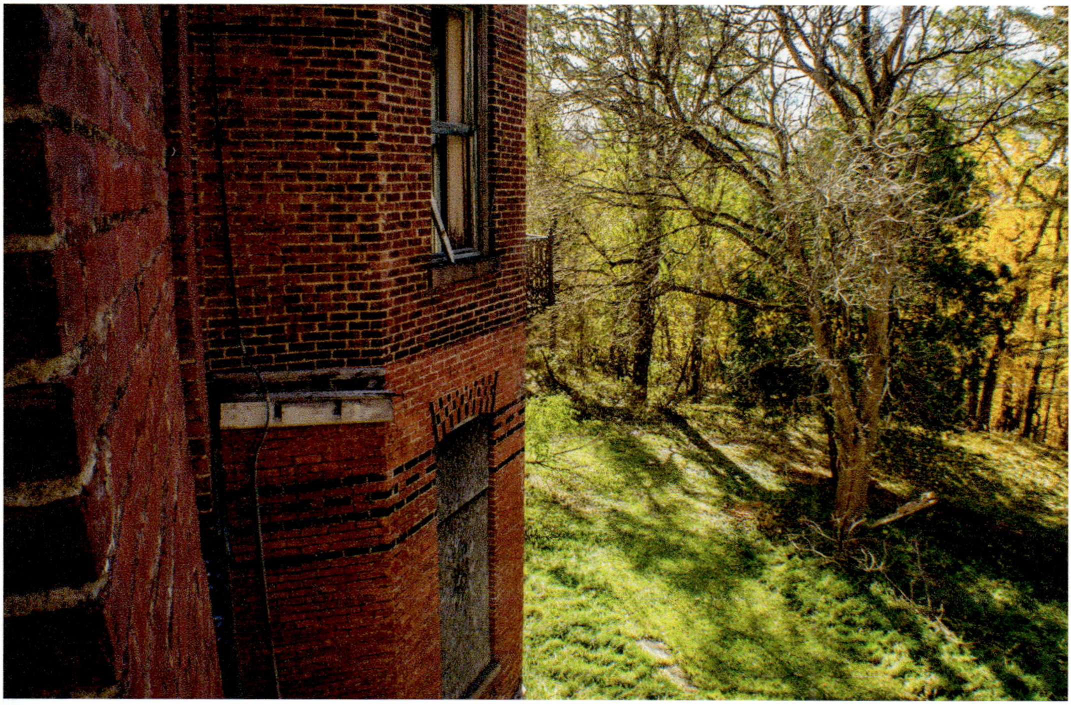

Deep red fades to rose as my eyes meet the embellished black patterns that wrap around the façade. As I peer out beyond the castle walls, I can only wonder what it felt like to stay here as an invalid. *[Photo by Brian Cray]*

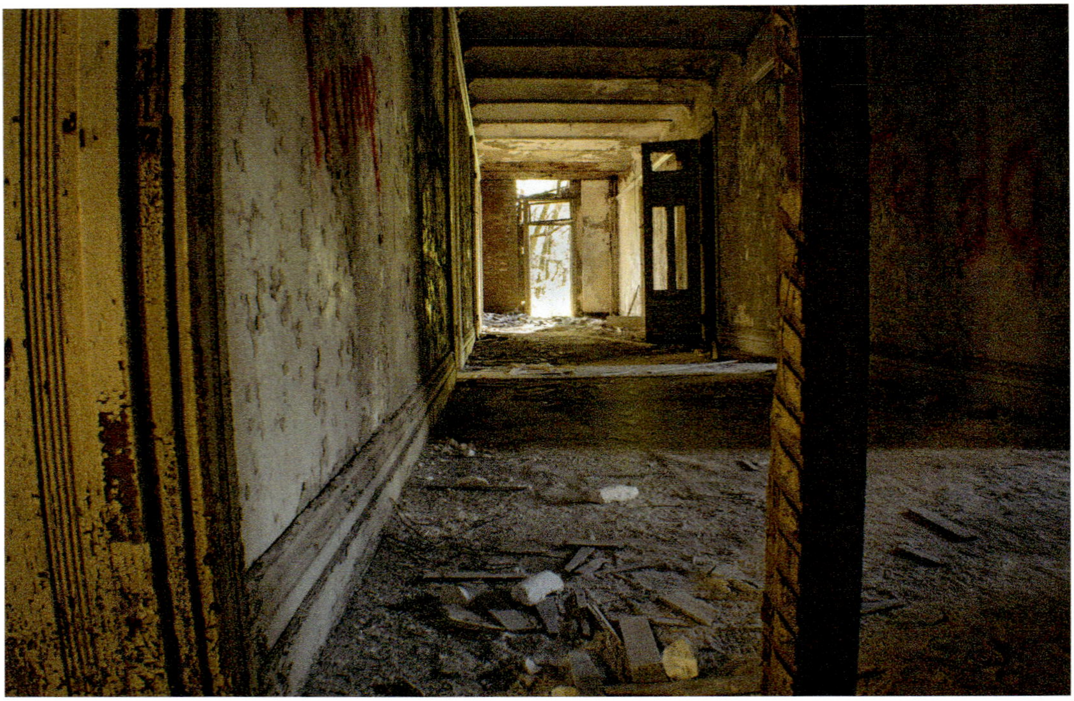

Brittle frames of splintered wood line the empty halls of dust and decay as I follow the sunlight to the crumbled ledge, which once connected to Liberty Hall. *[Photo by Brian Cray]*

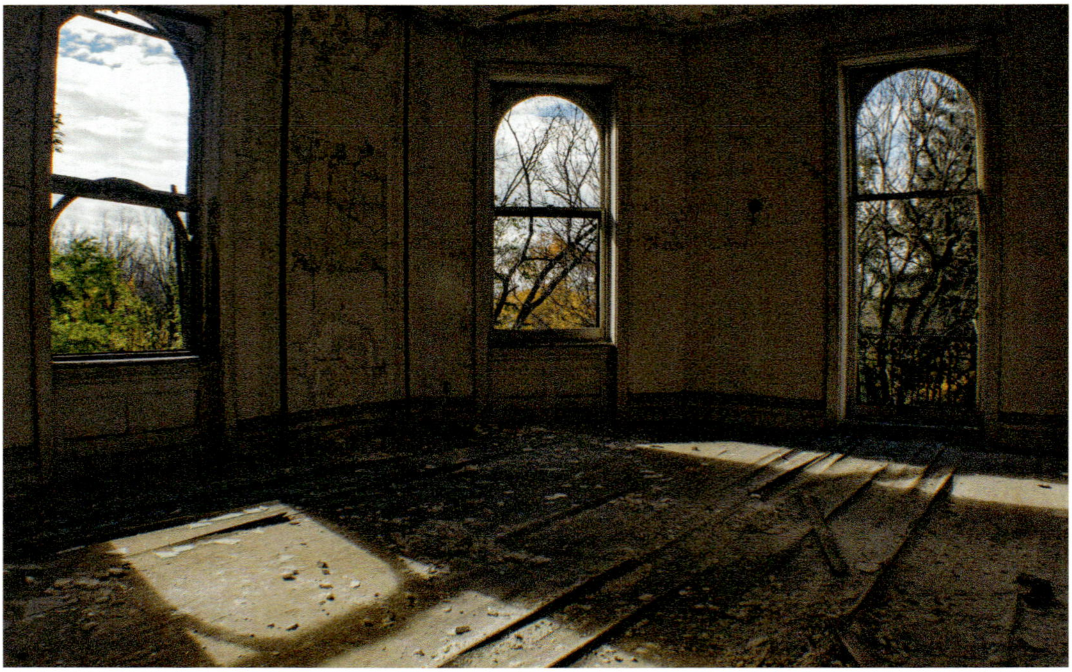

Even through years of decay, through winter storms, and relentless rain, majestic views permeate the windowpanes of every corner room. *[Photo by Brian Cray]*

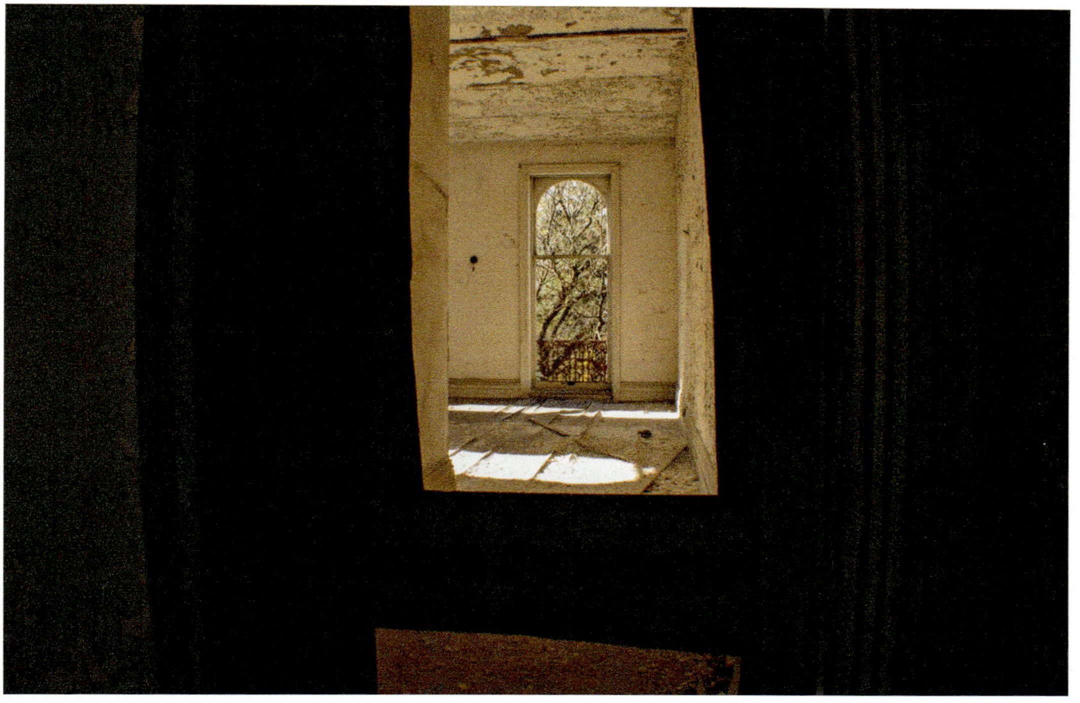

Dark split doorframes cannot hold back the thriving light of the forest. Nature will reclaim her land and soon will be forgotten. *[Photo by Brian Cray]*

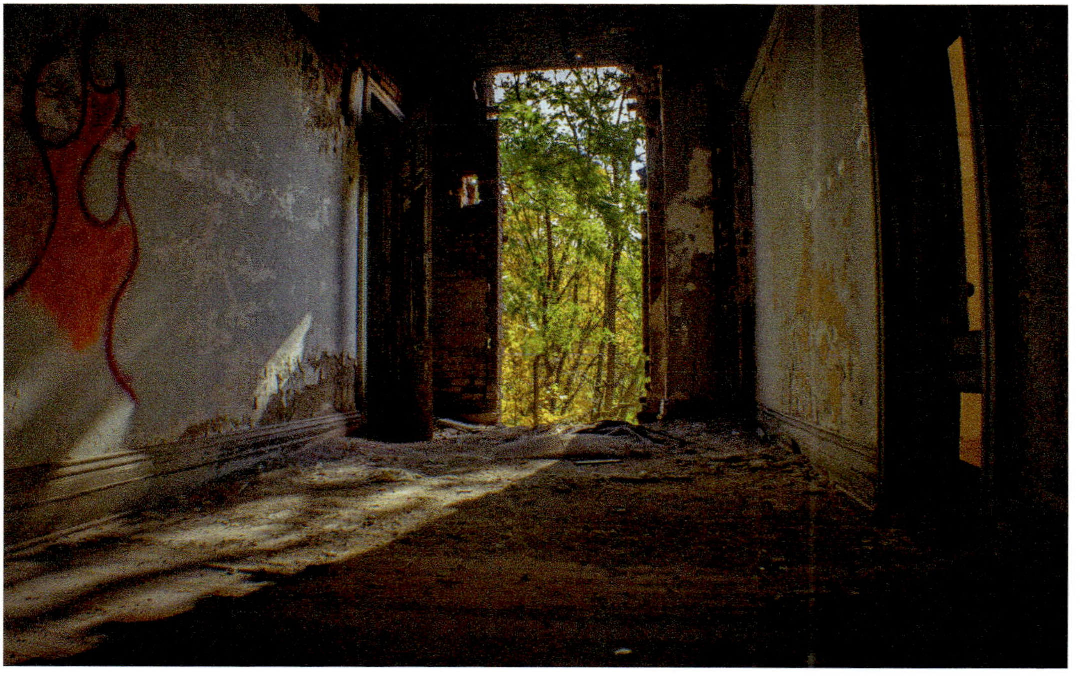

Through her flames light is born, but even Krog cannot revive her from her ashes. It has been too long. She is not a phoenix, but a fragile, old relic, and soon her pain will ease with time. *[Photo by Brian Cray]*

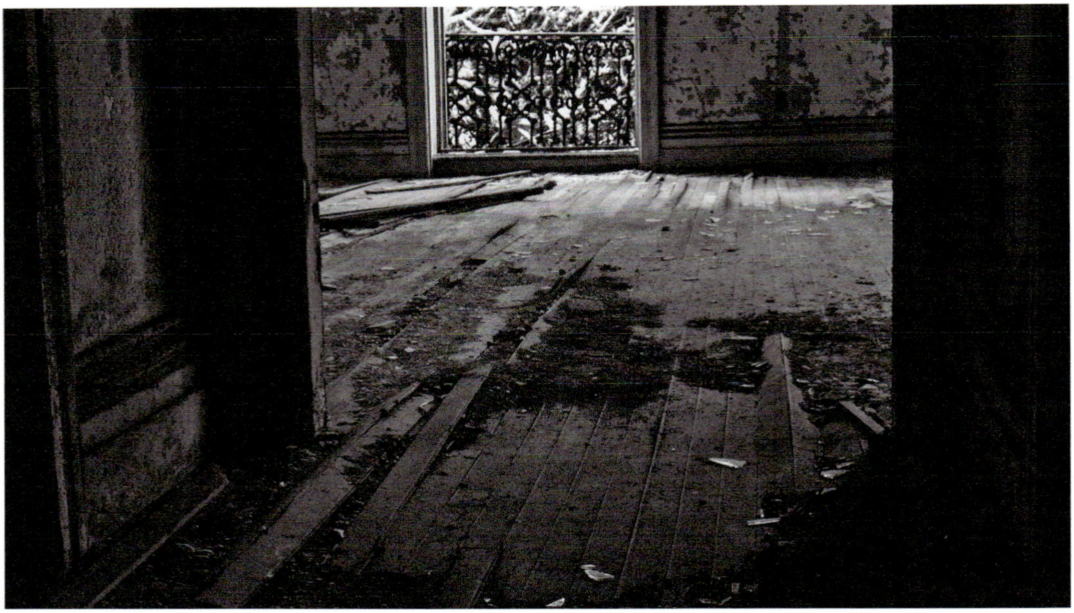

Distorted wood bends out of the floor like crooked teeth. Did you know Macfadden owned multiple sanatoriums throughout his lifetime? He opened one in the south side of Chicago called the Bernarr Macfadden Healthatorium. This $250,000 gothic-style mansion occupied a city block, standing five stories tall. (Adams, 2010) *[Photo by Brian Cray]*

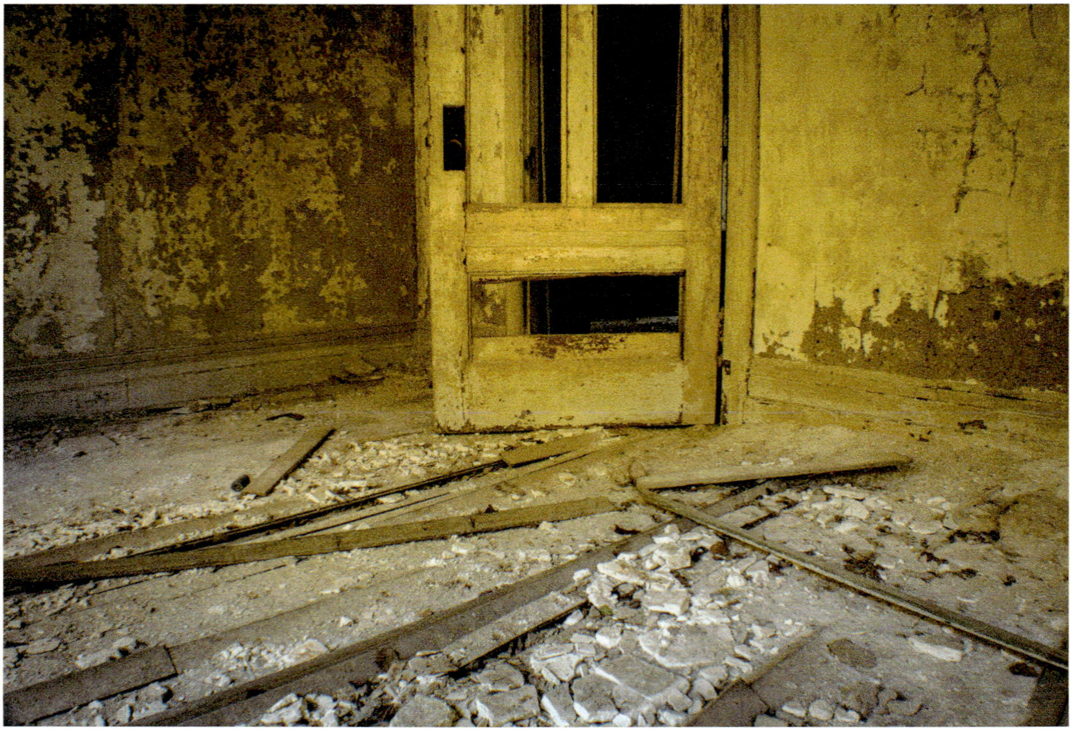

Every empty room looks so surreal if you haven't walked through her decrepit doors and felt the pain of her walls smeared amongst the floors. *[Photo by Brian Cray]*

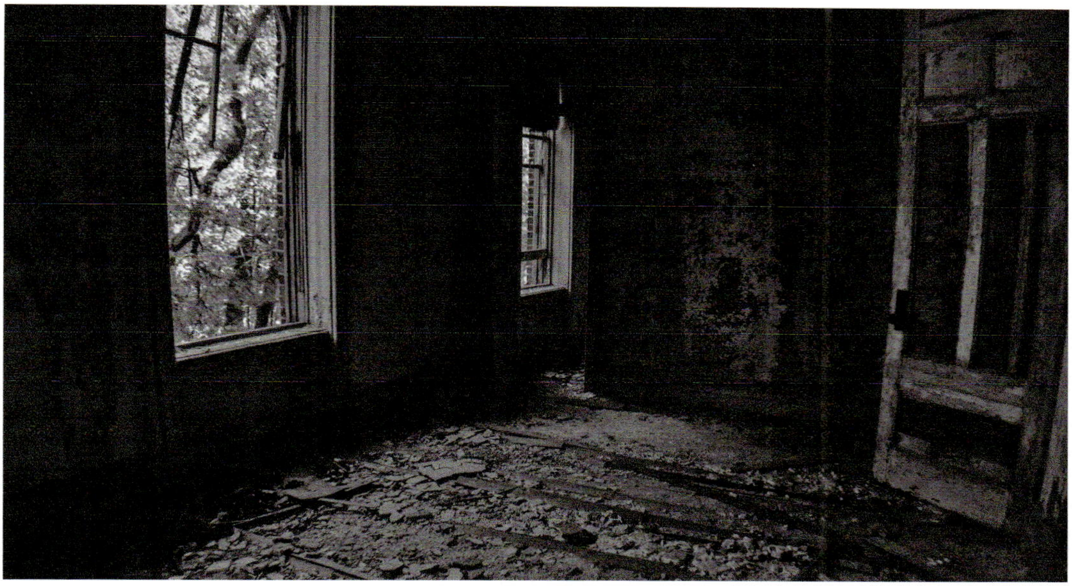

Macfadden ran Physical Culture Exhibitions to promote physical health, issuing contests for both men and women to show off their physique and test their athletic skills. Despite being a major success, he was arrested in 1905 for distribution of obscene photographs by Anthony Comstock and he was found guilty in 1906. (Adams, 2010) *[Photo by Brian Cray]*

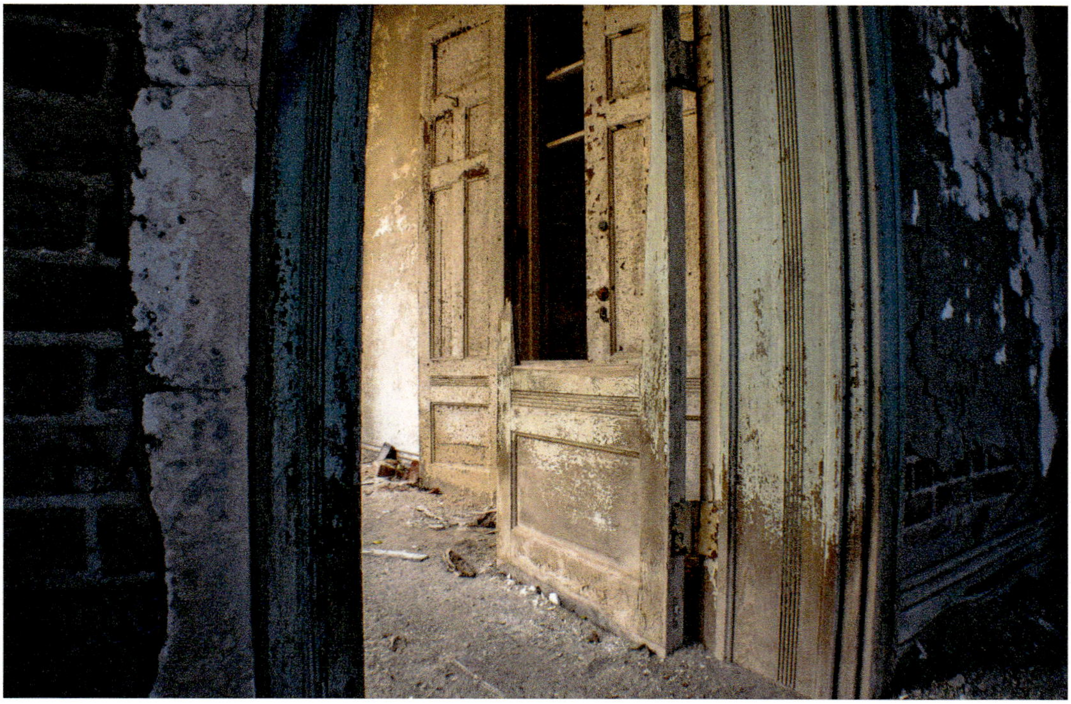

Mass production and shipping changed the accessibility of food in America and with it wrenched the epidemic of obesity, which in turn allowed entrepreneurs like Jackson and Macfadden to capitalize financially through diet and health regimens. (Adams, 2010) *[Photo by Brian Cray]*

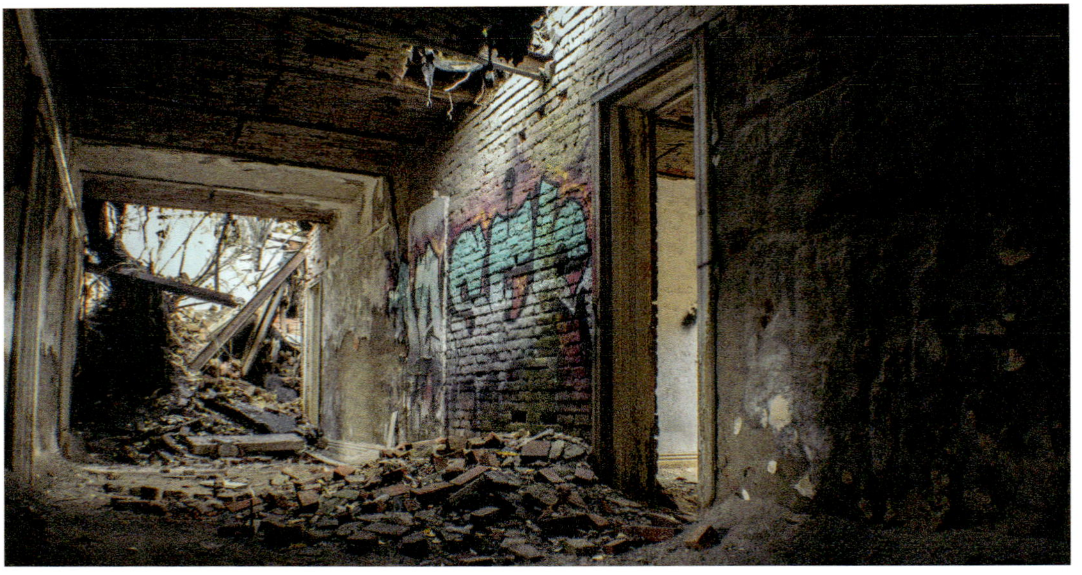

Bricks and steel beams teeter on the roof, decorating the floor in rubble, as the letters on the wall fade with the plague of decay. *[Photo by Brian Cray]*

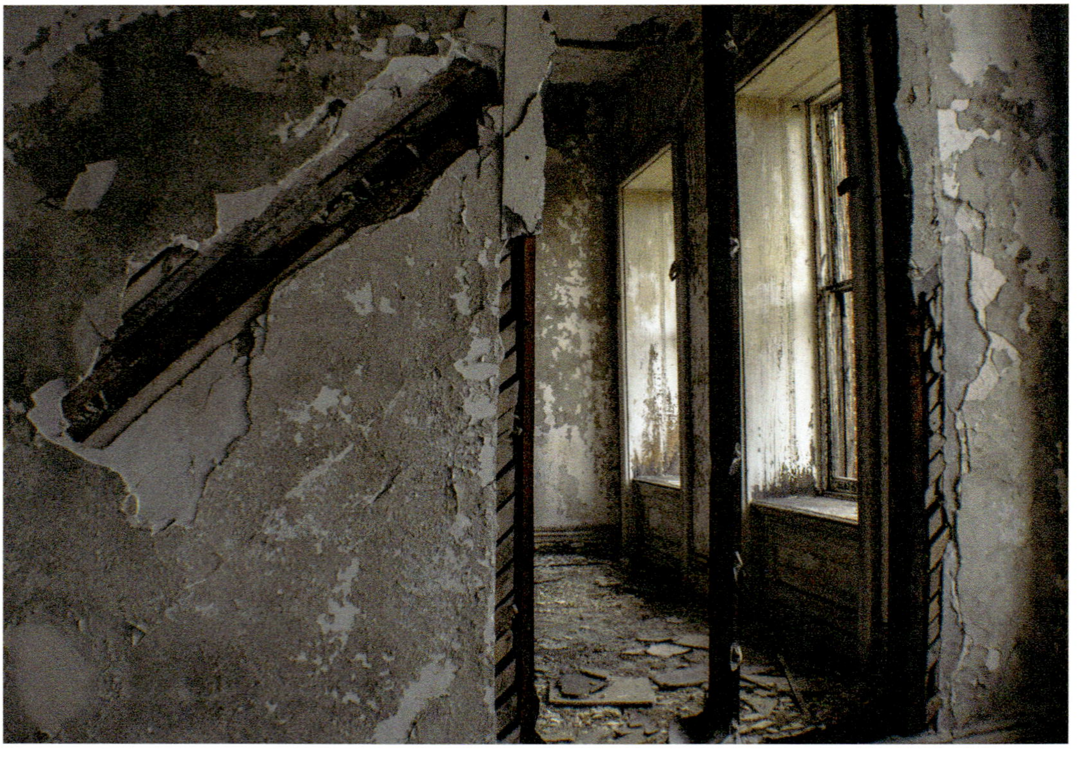

Empty rooms and barren walls, chips and scrapes of wooden blight, erase the past from crippling age. During its heyday, the institution was referred to as a great health institution rather than a "sanatorium" or "sanitarium." It was a safe haven for those seeking relaxation from nervous exhaustion and overwork, along with treating the invalid. *[Photo by Brian Cray]*

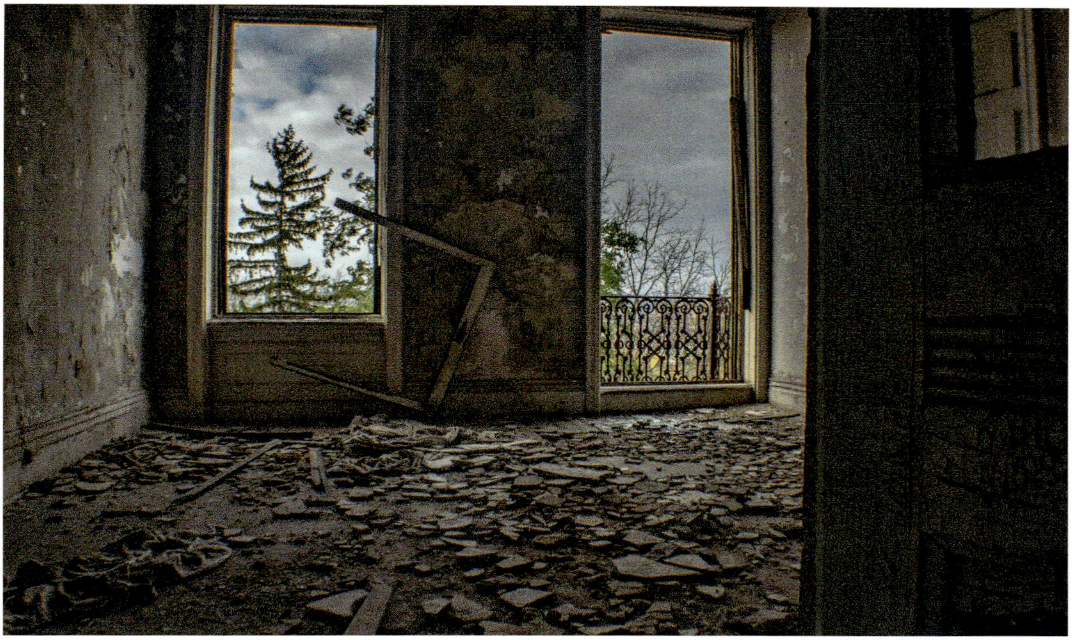

There is something about the chaos and disorder of each room that makes each picture feel like a surreal painting. Maybe it's the debris carpeting the floor. Maybe it's the perfectly titled window frame nestled against the wall. Maybe it's just beautiful decay? *[Photo by Brian Cray]*

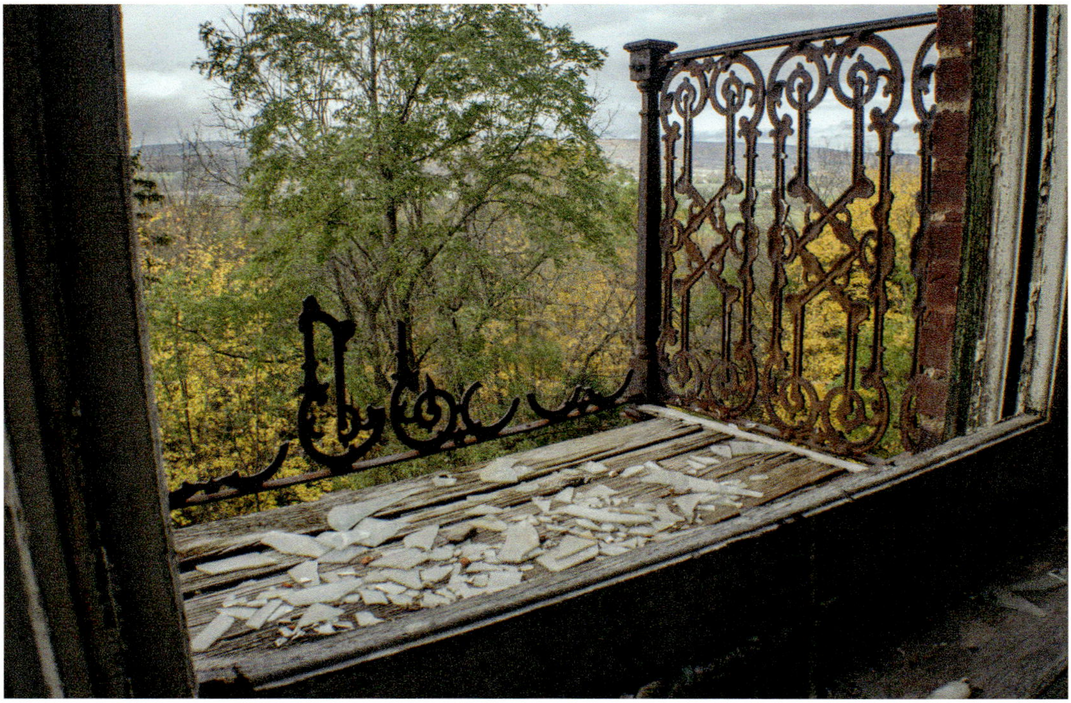

Roaring winds, pelting rain, drowning snow, fierce heat, and bone-chilling cold all ripped this baluster near its base. *[Photo by Brian Cray]*

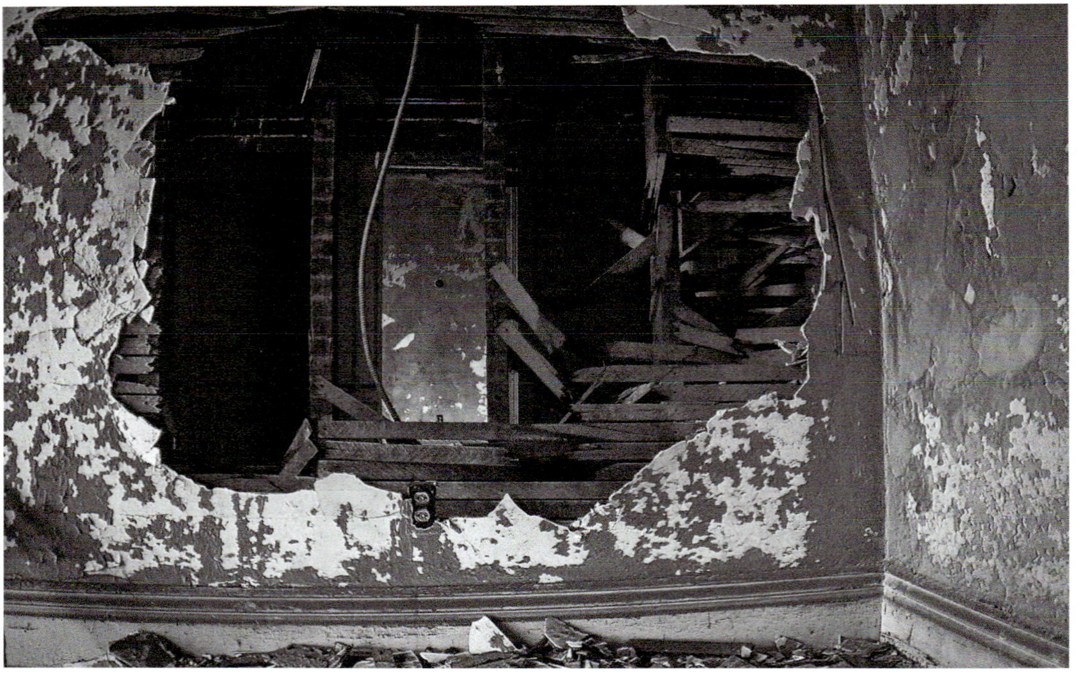

Smashed walls and busted wood act as multiple frames to an unusual picture as I trot closer to the rooftop, exploring each room. Macfadden published an encyclopedia of physical culture totaling 2,966 pages that detailed vegetarian recipes, sports and exercise, curing disease through physcultopathy, raw food diets and milk-based ones, fasting regimens, among expressing healthy views on sex. (Adams, 2010) *[Photo by Brian Cray]*

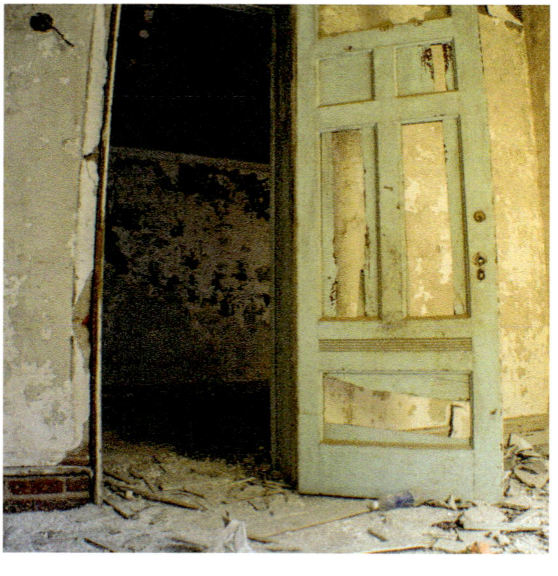

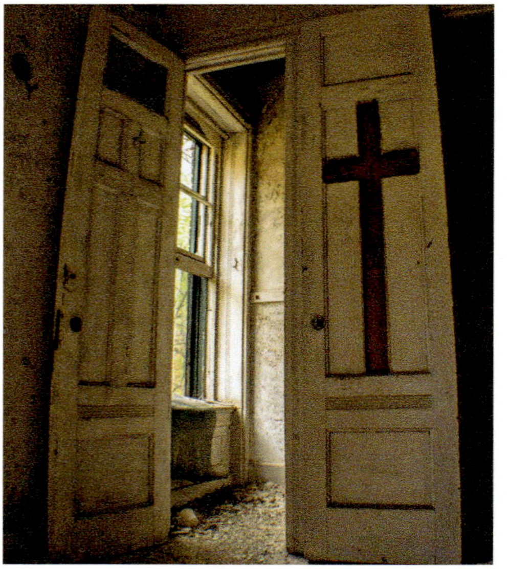

Above left: Every door looks the same as I wander room to room, looking at the jack-o-lantern smiles of wood, and the decay smeared across the floors in chunks of endless debris. *[Photo by Brian Cray]*

Above right: A cross parts the middle of the room waging war against good and evil. To the left is the path of light and to the right marks the path of darkness as Satan walks among the shadows. *[Photo by Brian Cray]*

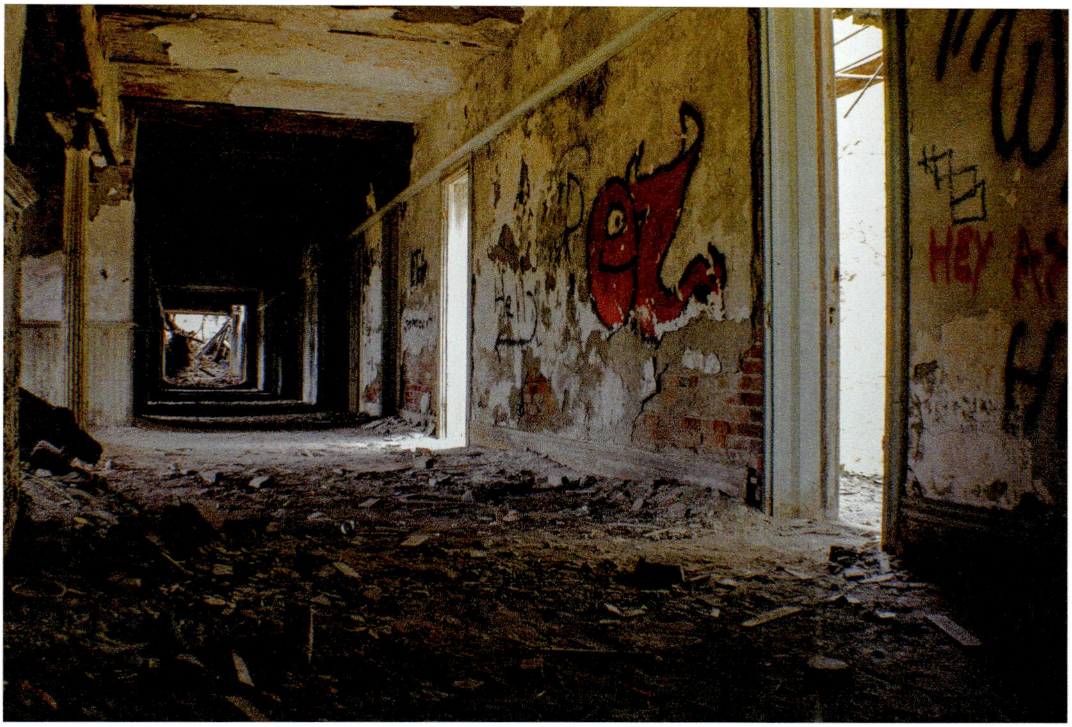

Behind the blistered walls of graffiti my eyes wander down the hallway, which feels almost infinite. Every door leads to nowhere. *[Photo by Brian Cray]*

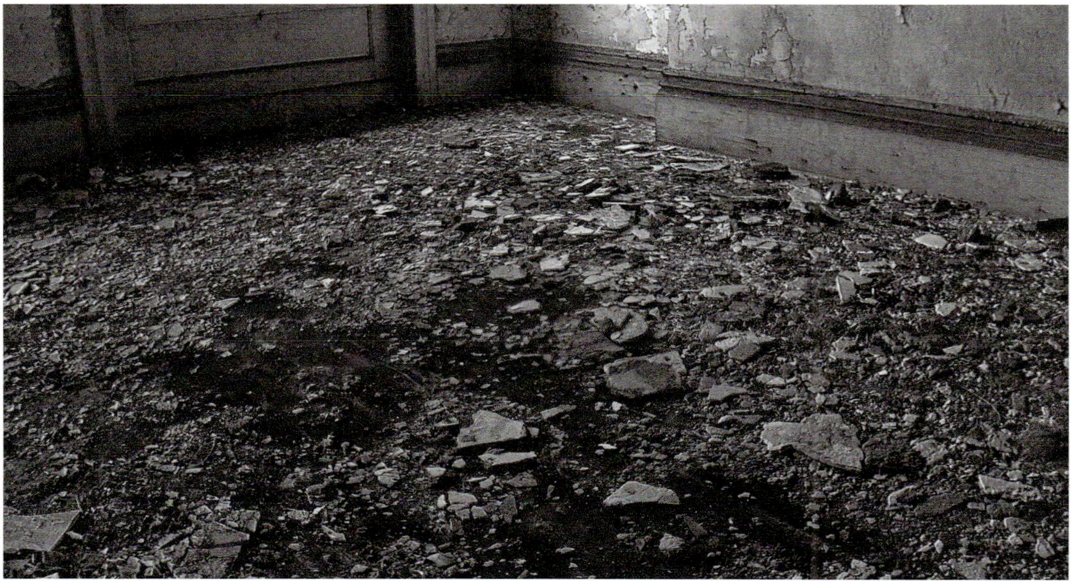

In the hopes of transplanting a utopian city just outside of Philadelphia and New York City, by the Pennsylvania Railroad, Macfadden purchased 1,800 acres in Spottswood to develop Physical Culture City. Two hundred faddists arrived that summer to adopt the physical culture lifestyle and vegetarian ways in fellowship setting. (Adams, 2010) *[Photo by Brian Cray]*

3

DAILY LIFE

A HISTORICAL ADAPTATION TO A TYPICAL DAY AT "THE SAN" IN THE 1860S

What was life like at the sanatorium? What did patients do on a typical day at "Our Home"? Well, according to Ted Jackson's *The Castles on the Hill,* it appears the daily routine followed a similar regimen to that of the Glen Haven facility.

Now close your eyes. Lay down on your bed. Wiggle your toes and free your mind of thought. Imagine you're a patient at "Our Home" and this is your story, a story similar to the diary of Elizabeth Walker, who attended "Our Home" in 1861-1862.

> It's morning. A twinkle of sunlight peels my eyelids open as it glares in through the arched window of my room. I ignore it and transgress back to a stupor, feeling quite sickly this morning like others, but suddenly, I flutter my eyes open as my ears ring to the resonating Chinese gong outside my door, the 6:00 a.m. wake-up call. I stiffly flounder about on my sea-grass mattress perched directly on slats and for the first time in nearly two weeks I unravel the chest jackets wrapping me tight like a mummy. I smile as I stand up. My bare feet tingle from the cool breath of wooden floor as I reach for my short dress (American Costume) in the closet. I feel free as it drapes loosely over my body like a night gown, unlike the wrenching grip of a corset, sinking its teeth into my ribcage like a vice.
>
> I stagger to open the door as my sweaty palms touch the brisk metal knob, sending quivering chills down my bony spine, making my heart sink in trepidation. I've lost nearly 7.5 lbs. in two weeks, but today Dr. Hurd will give me a new prescription for my pain as he mentioned yesterday during my examination. I slowly tiptoe into the hallway

as my wide eyes drift to the baluster, zigzagging to the ground floor, waiting for help down the stairwell. Mr. Layer and Mr. Schwan, employees of "Our Home," carry me downstairs as I sit in their arms like a chair. I make it just in time for Dr. Jackson's 7 a.m. lecture, in which he reiterates the importance of "not wasting energy in useless talk, thought and emotion." My spiritual journey wanders a sinuous path of ups and downs, but I know why I'm sick and it won't consume me. It won't! I pray daily, even if the doldrums lay me bedridden, depleted of all energy, unable to attend "Father's" sermon in the Chapel. It helps.

After Dr. Jackson's lecture on health, I wander down the corridor towards the dining room, peeking up at the Corinthian columns, chiseled with perfection. My eyes cast up at the architectural marvels wrapped around the interior, their strength, intricacies and beauty, and I hope one day I too will stand tall, fully restored to my previous health like the prowess of this building. As I sit down in the dining room, I hear the "mush" car creak through swing doors from the kitchen down the middle track like a freight car. The hot kettles atop it simmer like a steam engine and I wait for another serving of Graham Pudding with dates and graham crackers. They serve the 250 guests items off the healthiest of menus, packed together at each and every table, sitting on the newly upgraded wooden chairs from the previous stools they had just years prior.

We eat twice daily here. The food is plain, but they say pork will kill you, and I must say, I feel quite better since my change of diet. Grease no longer permeates my pores like viscous syrup and my gut rarely wrenches in pain, at least not like it used to anyway.

After breakfast, Dr. Hurd examines me between 10 a.m. and noon. He administers a Half Bath technique today, where I sit in six inches of water as his gentle hands rub my back and arms in a soothing massage while a nurse uses the same method upon my legs. Water splashes about over the course of two minutes, but afterwards I feel invigorated and ready for a sleigh ride with Dr. Jackson's son, Giles, along the east hillside. But first, they carry me back upstairs where I retire to a nice relaxing nap until 1:30 p.m. in my bedroom. I dream of playing backgammon and whist, dancing on the rooftop among the other guests, and all of the other fun activities.

As I grumble in pain, my eyes open after a feckless attempt to sleep. I still feel rested and excited for an hour and a half of free time. Giles knocks on my door and enters, helping me to my feet, and carries me down the steps for an outdoor sleigh ride along the hill. Christmas trees, draped in fluffy white snow, droop along the rolling hillside up to the railroad tracks as he pulls me around outside the wooden edifice. I smile and laugh. The resort truly feels like family here, but I fear that I will not be able to attend dinner this evening due to sudden exhaustion. Staff carry me up to my room where I eat boiled rice, green peas, and barely nibble into my potato biscuits. Free time lasts until 8:30 p.m., but tonight, instead of playing backgammon or whist, I will take a gander off the piazza and watch the sun dip below the clouds, relishing in the bright fire painted endlessly across the Dansville sky. For up here in this castle, you can see clear across the Genesee Valley and it almost feels timeless, as if the pain stops for a second like nature's cure. Once the curtains of night infect the sky with a field of fireflies, I scurry back to my bed for another night's rest before dipping into another day at "Our Home" in the 1860s.[1]

4

THE LION'S ROAR

A Brief History on Bernarr Macfadden and the Physical Culture Hotel

After the Jackson Health Resort declared bankruptcy in 1914 and completely abandoned its operation in 1917, it changed hands multiple times, acting as a psychiatric hospital for World War I veterans suffering from PTSD, along with going through a plethora of feckless owners whom could not get it off the ground as a health resort.[1] That all changed with the lion's roar when eccentric businessman, Bernard McFadden, relocated to Dansville and opened a "healthatorium."

Born as Bernard Aldophus McFadden in Mill Springs, Missouri, a small town in the Ozarks, on August 16, 1868, he spent his early years as a poor, feeble child with a rough and lonely upbringing on a farm along the Black River.[2] With a father who exhausted his farm earnings on corn whiskey and betting the ponies, his profligate addictions and inebriation led him to beat his family.[3] It was only a matter of time before Bernard's mother left for her parents in Ironton, escaping the plague of abuse with her two youngsters.[4] Not long after, Bernard's father died within the year of their separation from delirium tremens.[5] Once Bernard recovered from a six-month painful scuffle with smallpox (this led to his hatred of vaccinations), his deathly ill mother, suffering from tuberculosis, sent him off to the only boarding school she could afford.[6] Bernard kicked and screamed, grazing at his mother's arms as an employee of the orphan school dragged him along the wharf to a steamship, sending him off down the Mississippi River to starvation academy. His malnourished classmates enlightened him with a juicy tidbit, "They never feed us *nothin'* here."[7] Bernard spent a year there consuming more whole peanuts than he would in his elder years when he trained for the circus.

Soon after his ninth birthday, his mother arranged a work-trade opportunity for him in Mount Sterling, Illinois, with her distant relatives who owned a cheap hotel, in which Bernard worked 100-hour weeks for room and board.[8] This lasted up until her death in 1879 from tuberculosis, which left Bernard an orphan.[9] He hopped from home to home, where he landed on Farmer Macomb's doorstep in exchange for produce and a small lump sum of cash before trickling over to Farmer Hunter where he learned the importance of physical strength and health, shown through his calloused hands and whimpering bones.[10, 11] After many days' work of shucking corn, gathering sap, churning butter, and tending to cattle, among his other daily household chores, his meager skeleton frame morphed into a brawny little Hercules.[12] The kids in town that once picked on him as a feeble weakling now succumbed to his strength and his name, the "terrible good fighter," resonated amongst them.[13]

He climbed the many rungs to adulthood in his early years through his hard work, performing the same tasks as an adult farmhand, but receiving little more than room and board for compensation, with not even a new pair of boots to keep his toes from freezing during the harsh winter.[14] So he left the only way he knew how, by walking two miles into town and then hopped a train, adopting a short-lived, footloose lifestyle as a penniless wanderer looking for his next gig as he shuffled through extended family.[15]

Once he reached St. Louis, after years as an unwanted orphan and child slave laborer on two separate farms, he finally saddled up in the fruitful home of his uncle Harvey P. Miller, taking a job with Dun and Co. as a delivery boy before moving up to an office position at his uncle's grocery store.[16] Life looked promising and hopeful despite his bleak past, which had left him bloodied and bruised from his father's raging outbursts, emaciated from eating peanuts (shells and all) at the cheapest of boarding schools, and emotionally blistered without parents and in the hands of people who neglected him.[17] But the brittle winter of 1882-1883 marked his deepest troubles as he fought difficulties with his health, trying useless remedies and placebo medicines with little to no effect on his well-being.[18] He dropped to a meager 100 pounds and revelation struck him like an angel.[19]

From that moment forward, he never let the events of his past affect his future endeavors as not only a successful entrepreneur and a pioneer of physical fitness, but as an aspiring strongman. He purged the harsh words of his conscience that muttered "consumption" and vowed for a different path, not defined by predestination, but by free will. He wanted to come out swinging, with muscles and force, and choose his own life, which did not include the likes of "alcohol, tobacco, white bread, meat, or even medicine."

He yearned for strength, fortitude, and purpose. That day when he walked by the Missouri Gymnasium with his uncle and nephew, locked his eyes on the sculpted physiques of living statues, pumping iron and grunting loudly under strain, changed him for life.[20] He wanted to look just like them. He wanted the grip of a gorilla and the chiseled body of a lion, so he scrounged money together and spent fifty cents on second-hand dumbbells.[21] That night he commenced his own weight training program and never looked back.

As his strength increased, his bulging muscles demanded more weight, so he purchased heavier dumbbells, on top of walking six miles to and from work with a ten-pound lead bar in his shirt.[22] He strove for perfect masculinity. With his roots like stone in regular physical activity, it was not until he explored the vast realm of dietary options that he truly embodied the basis for physical culture in America. As a young teenager he stumbled upon the works of Sylvester Graham, and much like James Caleb Jackson, Bernard fostered his own ideologies on "health food," abstaining from caffeinated beverages, red meat, and white bread, and vocalizing the importance of his unorthodox diet in his later lectures as an adult.[23]

As a teenager still finding his place in the world, he took to the rails, bumming around after city life burdened him with monotony.[24] He set out for Kansas at sixteen, where his cousin, Medearis, started a dentistry outpost.[25] He shuffled back and forth between throwing patients in headlocks for tooth extraction and working as a farmhand for ten dollars a week plus meals.[26] But his gypsy blood and palpable spirit cursed him and he switched professions yet again, dabbling at teaching boxing in a horse stable and working on a local newspaper with his cousin, called the *McCune Brick*.[27] Both of these flopped horrendously with no financial gains, and so he returned to St. Louis.[28]

At the ripe age of seventeen, he stood firmly with his decision to pursue physical culture as a career as his boisterous attitude, baseball-sized biceps, and whole life revolved around it. When Bernard was not bookkeeping for his Uncle Harvey, you could find him flexing his muscles at the Missouri Gymnasium, finally having saved enough money to enter it, in tights and a sleeveless shirt.[29] He loved the throbbing pump of adrenaline flowing through his veins and a rampant heartbeat that sang success. Nothing beat that euphoric feeling of becoming god-size after an intense session of picking things up and putting them down. He worked out with his Greek-American friend George Baptiste.[30]

With weight lifting, he naturally stumbled into an unknown ambition to pursue wrestling, where he switched his dietary regimen to two meals a day. He would go on to preach this for the rest of his life as he deemed lower-caloric intake and borderline starvation were the cure for any sickness. At least once or twice, his anorexic experiments drove him too close to starvation, causing him to faint and suffer severe dehydration and jaundice—nonetheless that did not stop him from such extremism.[31]

It was at eighteen he discovered his loud-mouthed talent of attracting an audience through a natural gift of public outreach and promotion. He utilized this skill to compete with some of the top athletes in the nation in wrestling tournaments, boosting his ego and increasing his pockets as he battled with the insecurities of his name, which he later changed to Bernarr Macfadden for a more masculine touch with the zing of a lion's roar on the "R."[32]

But all of this attention and physical perfection did not fulfill Bernarr's thirst for stardom; he needed more, but what else was there? He wanted to stitch the wounds of his fledgling education or lack thereof so he churned in the books, instead of the butter as a farmhand, or the weights as a fitness enthusiast, to garner the skills required to VOICE his philosophies in comprehensible language for everyone to read. And that year, in 1891, he crafted a sign, which became his first steps to becoming a successful, renowned man. It read:

> BERNARD MCFADDEN – KINISITHERAPIST
> TEACHER OF HIGHER PHYSICAL CULTURE

With no actual dictionary definition existing for "kinisitherapist," he figured it witty enough to attract attention of passersby in order to employ his art of physical culture to tackle disease through exercise and movement. It did for a while, and he lived quite comfortably, but as he tweaked his high-fiber diet to find his sweet spot, he binged on copious exercise regimens, and further starved his body of calories. This deflected his digestive problems, while destroying his physique, and he looked like the epitome of anorexia, scaring off any clientele he once garnered through his creative ploys.[33]

Through many years, and a great deal of failures, Bernarr exhausted time and funds, and worked undoubtedly hard to propel himself to fame, never giving up and always gunning forward, striving for success. He did not concern himself much with fortune, but yearned for remembrance and for voice and purpose in his life.

In his twenties, with the repertoire of skills he acquired from hustling and tramping around America as an adolescent, trying to capitalize on obscure niches to make a buck, he found himself lacking key elements in grammar and writing structure to become successful. In order to launch his platform of physical culture to the world, he enrolled in Bunker Hill Military Academy to master literature in hopes of publishing his rejected articles. In exchange for his labor, he received an education and room and board to master literacy, spending a year at the academy before returning to hustling wrestling bouts for a living, which earned him champion titles for all weight divisions in Chicago.[34] He capitalized off his notoriety until it faded away and he leapt to his next stint of unconventional endeavors.

He found himself wandering back to St. Louis, where he dipped into coaching football and wrestling at Marmaduke, while writing his first 80,000-word novel, *The Athlete's Conquest*, a bizarre fictional portrayal of a young man's quest to find a loving bride of physical culture. No publisher would consider it, referring to it as "crude junk," but that did not stop Bernarr from revising it and distributing it amongst the students of Marmaduke.[35]

Many of his endeavors ended with little financial success, but Bernarr never capitulated to failure—instead, it drove him to keep plugging away at new ideas until one came to fruition. He stowed ideas away from the strength success of body-sculpting phenomenon, Eugen Sandow. Sandow earned a respectable income posing as a muscular masterpiece with only a leaf covering his appendage as he flexed his godlike temple for the masses. He also published a magazine strictly focused on physical fitness called *Physical Culture,* which he released in England.[36]

Then the lion's roar emerged loud enough for all to hear from Manhattan to England. What started off as Bernarr hustling semi-naked, risqué photographs similar to the works of Sandow, which he had seen at the World Fair in Chicago, landed him on a boat to England, preaching bodybuilding, with demonstrations of his exercise programs and lectures on physical culture.[37]

His performances copied Sandow's presentations almost identically, but he capitalized more on them in England than in America.[38] In fact, he collected all his rejected blurbs and articles, publishing bits and pieces in a brochure for his exerciser program, which led to huge success. This manual of physical fitness began to grow to an encyclopedia-sized volume of physical culture and manifested popularity quite quickly, skyrocketing Macfadden to both fame and fortune. In the world of health, he would name it *Physical Culture*, the same name of Sandow's magazine in England that was released a year prior.[39]

His magazine separated from the norm as he plowed head first into crude topics of sex, celebrity gossip, physical culture, and diet, and was complemented by risqué cosmographs, with his message targeted to both genders. Women revered him as a feminist and many of his followers deemed him a god among men. His sales soared to the moon, reeling in 25,000 copies by January of 1900. They featured writings by the likes of Sandow, Charles Eliot, and John Sullivan and covered unorthodox topics promoting vegetarianism, bodybuilding, anti-vaccination, and diet.[40]

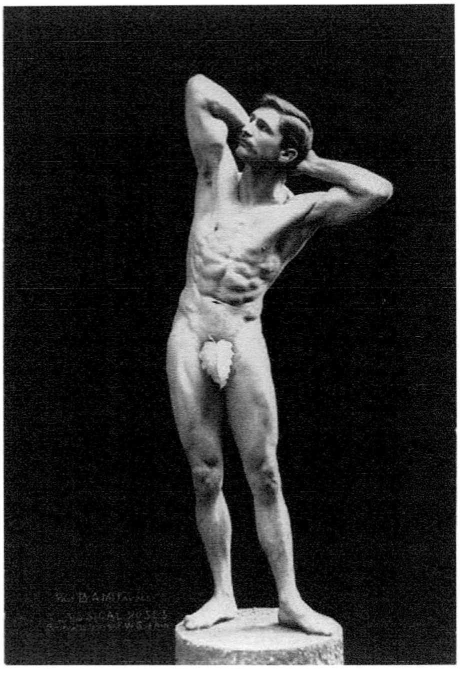

This is one of Macfadden's many poses with a fig leaf, which he conveniently copied off of bodybuilder Eugen Sandow and was able to capitalize off of it in not one, but two continents, which brought him huge success for his publishing empire. *[Photo catalogued by Library of Congress]*

After just the first few years, sales skyrocketed to 110,000 copies per month and profits totaled $90,000.[41] Bernarr transformed himself from a street hustling hooligan to a publishing prodigy and became known as one of the leading experts in physical health as he revolutionized the world of journalism for generations to come. In total, his publishing empire sold close to 50 million copies of the magazine between the world wars.[42] He would later go on to publish *True Story Magazine* in 1919 and *The Graphic* in 1924, which gained negative criticism as the *Pornographic* for its obscene cosmographs, but all were considered financially successful for Macfadden and he kept scribbling away, printing books, magazines and newspapers and becoming one of the most successful publishers in America.[43] He had made a name for himself, not just in New York, but nationwide. *Time Magazine* even recognized his feats, coining him "Body Love" Macfadden, and with countless ties to the publishing world, and a boatload of peculiarities that added to a seemingly endless résumé, Macfadden dipped into other new endeavors as a renowned public icon.[44]

He opened a string of chains called the Physical Culture Restaurant, which provided options for vegetarians, and marketed huge success, operating multiple venues in New York, Boston, Philadelphia and Chicago.[45] Over the next twenty years he held bodybuilding competitions, exercised like a maniac, continued his strict diet regimen, attended to his daily publishing duties, and opened multiple health spas in Long Island, Battle Creek, and the south side of Chicago, to name a few, all of which never lasted too long and not nearly as long as his baby in Dansville, anyway. He actually swore he would never run such an institution again, but we all know Macfadden now.[46] He just can't take no for an answer. He won't give up and wave his white flag. Nope!

In 1929, he purchased the Jackson Health Resort, renaming it to Bernarr Macfadden's Hotel and later changing its name to the Physical Culture Hotel.[47] The health spa promoted long walks, naked sunbathing on the roof, water cure, spinal strengthening, fasting and the milk diet while he also employed specialized MD personnel, trained in natural methods for treatment of "anemia, asthma, auto-intoxication, catarrh, constipation, diabetes, heart diseases, influenza, insomnia, obesity, cerebral palsy, rheumatism, stomach diseases, thinness among a slew of other non-contagious ailments."[48]

Macfadden's principles on diet and physical health rallied against the accepted medical practices of that era and his cultist ideas opposed drugs, deeming them "poison." He had learned from a young age never to trust them, leaving him blood poisoned for six months, fighting smallpox and painfully suffering on his death bed with lung fever without much relief. His blood boiled at the mere mentioning of "drugs" and from it he stemmed the seven pillars that cursed humanity:[49]

Prudishness
Corsets
Muscular Inactivity
Gluttony
Drugs
Alcohol
Tobacco

Bernarr's reign in Dansville transitioned the water cure facility to a recreational spa fit for individuals looking for extreme body transformations, pain relief, and cures to sicknesses, among just "getting away from it all." Aside from the plethora of physical activities and training regimens in place for patrons to lose weight or rid their bodies of illnesses were the sponsored "Cracked Wheat Derbies." Macfadden took forty-eight hikers, aged nineteen to eighty-three, in a 325-mile walkathon from Dansville to New York City just to prove that the human body could survive two weeks on a diet solely consisting of cracked wheat rather than potatoes and steak.[50] It completely rebuilt people, reshaping their bodies and trimming their frames, boosting their energy levels and self-esteem.

Like thunder ruminating in the clouds, Bernarr's creed to physical culture recognized weakness as not only a menace, but a crime. He preached about the virility to superb health and manliness in the many brochures plastered throughout the Physical Culture Hotel (the P.C.). He touted fresh air and sunlight, thorough mastication of wholesome foods with a day or two of fasting, routine muscular activity, frequent bathing for cleanliness and cleansing, and maintaining a powerful mind as the key to becoming a perfectly sculpted specimen of extraordinary health.[51] He believed the hotel was the largest of its kind and the most progressive in the world because it taught practices built on the foundations of his physcultopathy.[52]

The P. C. received 200 patrons each summer and Macfadden stressed that it was not a sanitarium, nor did they accept contagious, venereal, tubercular, or mental patients into his institution.[53, 54] Instead, they accepted patients with common ailments. The P. C. built its principles off of the five "Rs" to regain one's health to normal levels:[55]

Restoration
Rebuilding
Rest
Recreation
Rehab

Gravity boards, sun ray lamps, electric and steam cabinets, along with Moliere, Nauheim, Sitz, Brine, Aix and Scotch douches all aimed to rest and soothe the body back to its invigorated form.[56] Most patients basked in Swedish Massages, undergoing salt, ice, oil, or alcohol rubs.[57] Macfadden encouraged guests to sunbathe in the nude on the towers at the ends of the roof that were separated by gender. Patrons walked the myriad hillside trails among the 30-acres of dense forest when not dancing on the rooftop, attending his morning exercise classes, or engaging in the other activities offered by the resort, which were also encouraged.[58] A recommended eight- to twelve-week stay was suggested per patron to completely rid the body of toxins and revitalize them to complete health.[59] Upon entering the facility, one received a physical examination by a licensed physician of New York State. One met with a physician on a daily basis as he monitored progress while issuing the proper prescriptions of diet, massage, baths, and exercise. These methods, in full force, healed! The health building courses held in the auditorium also administered valuable information to enforce mental toughness in patrons. Depression did NOT exist at the P. C.: only cheer and a precious desire for a healthy life. Bernarr lived by this and preached these methods for well over forty years.[60]

When he wasn't preaching or fighting random passersby, Bernarr hunted attention and publicity as much as he sculpted his physique, appearing countless times in magazines, newspapers and published works, symbolizing the first Mr. America.

His thirst for fame never quenched his ego and even with age he never capitulated to failure. Instead, he garnered it to further endorse his beliefs by touting low-fat diet, constant exercise, power walking, and reiterating time and time again that "medicine is poison." How did he do this? On one occasion, for his eighty-third birthday, he performed a low-altitude static-line jump out of a Stinson monoplane, landing on his back on the sandy New Jersey shoreline by the Hudson.[61] He stood up, brushing the sand off his goofy getup—which consisted of a football helmet, red flannel underwear and life jacket—as reporters huddled around him to flaunt his age-defying stunt.[62] Macfadden, a genius entrepreneur, invited the lot back to his dwelling to boast not his recent skydive, but the importance of health, hygiene, and exercise to the longevity of life. His employment of such philosophies not only educated the world, but his stubbornness that followed such views led to his ultimate demise, and he vanished like a speck in the sky by eighty-five, not from a malfunctioning reserve parachute, but from an untreated urinary tract infection.[63]

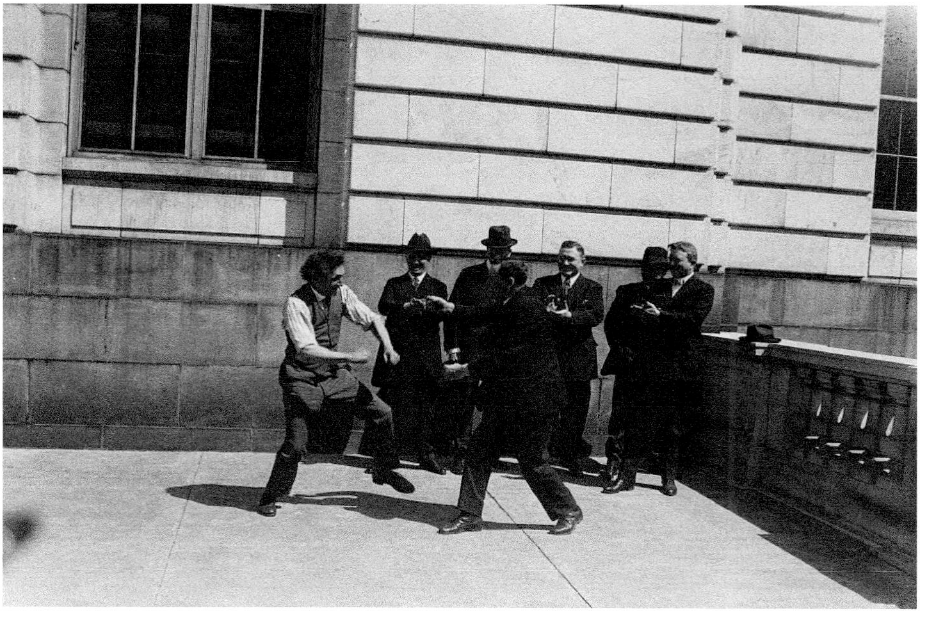

It was not uncommon to see the eccentric Macfadden bare-knuckle boxing in public. In this photo, he is roughhousing with Senator Smith W. Brookhart of Iowa outside of the senator office building. *[Harris & Ewing, photographer]*

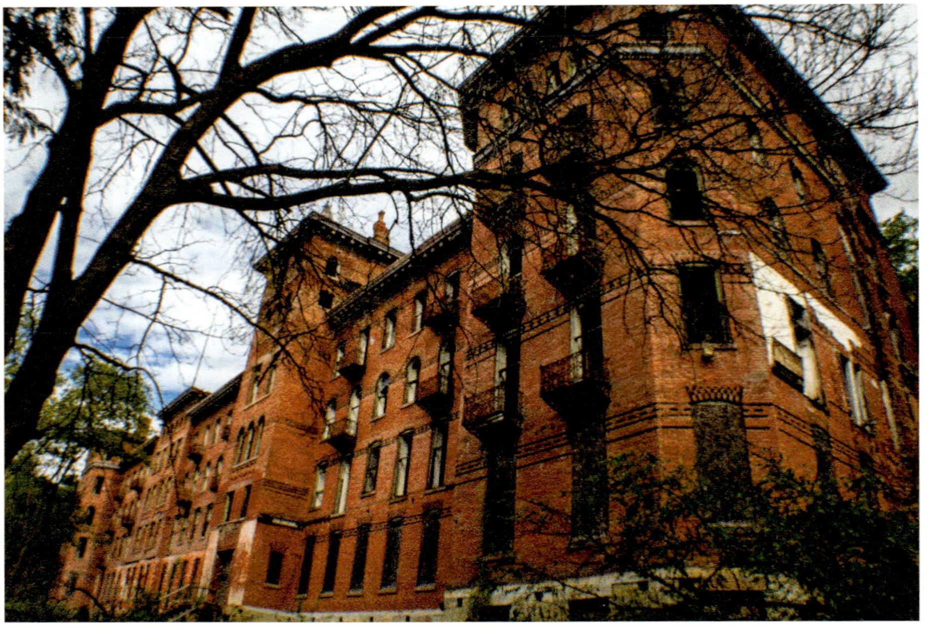

Despite dying at twenty-nine from consumption, Giles E. Jackson left behind his legacies of designing and constructing Liberty Hall, which is where health lectures, religious services and entertainments took place. *[Photo by Brian Cray]*

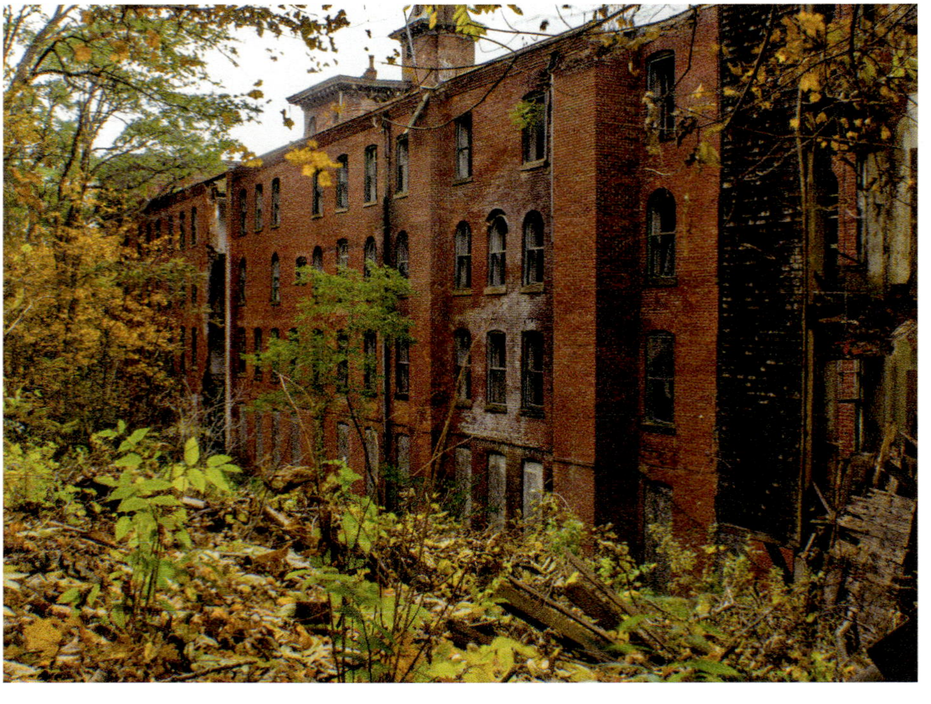

Creeping through the back woods, I peer out at the castle standing like a delicate flower with heaps of rubble at her base beyond the autumn leaves, through jagged scars lay splintered wood, stray bricks, warped steel beams and rusted pipes. *[Photo by Brian Cray]*

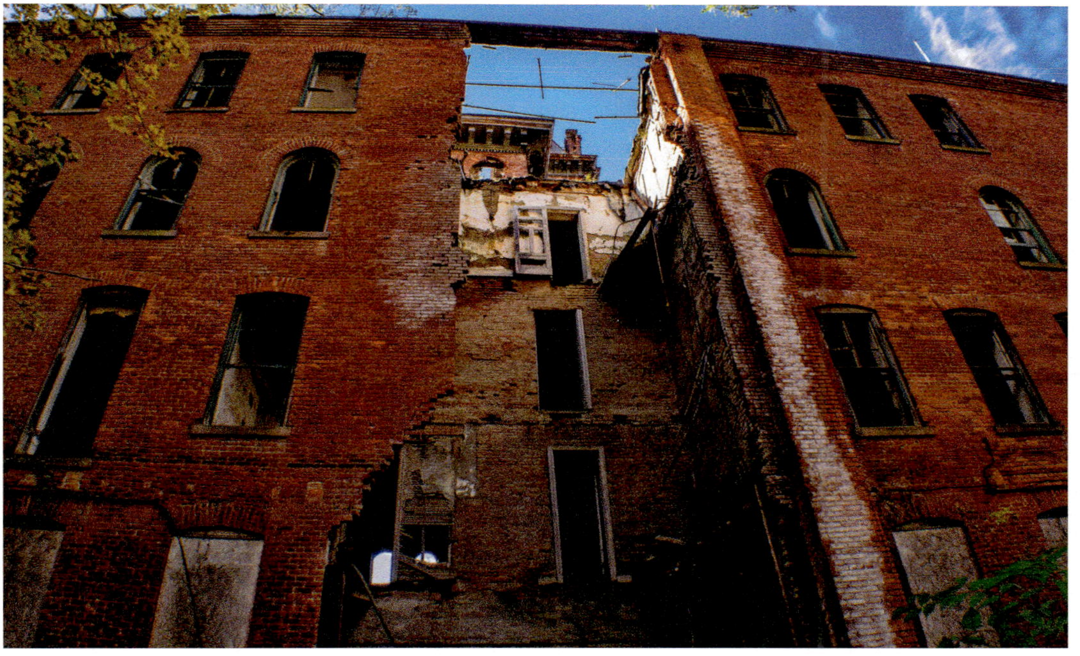

Toothed brick severs away from the back red façade like the missing piece to a jigsaw puzzle, and a clear view of the gouged roof sits in my mind through the bluest of skies. *[Photo by Brian Cray]*

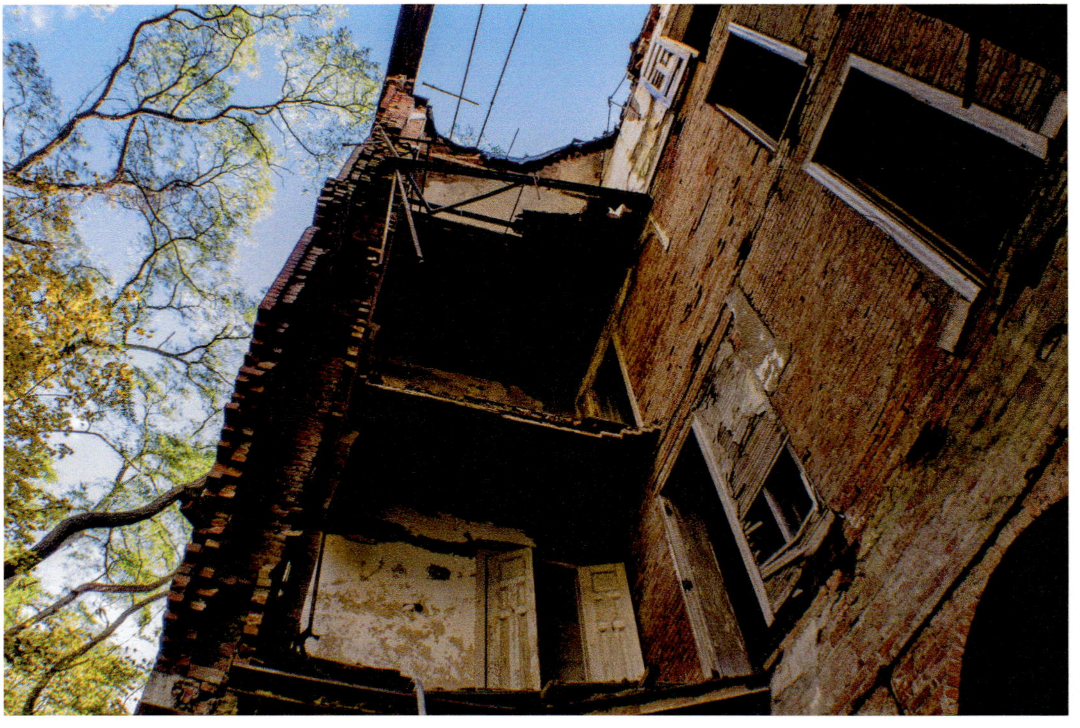

Jagged bricks descend from the roof, opening holes to rooms of distant memories. Somewhere beneath this rubble are pieces of the reception area, the second-floor solarium and guest rooms. *[Photo by Brian Cray]*

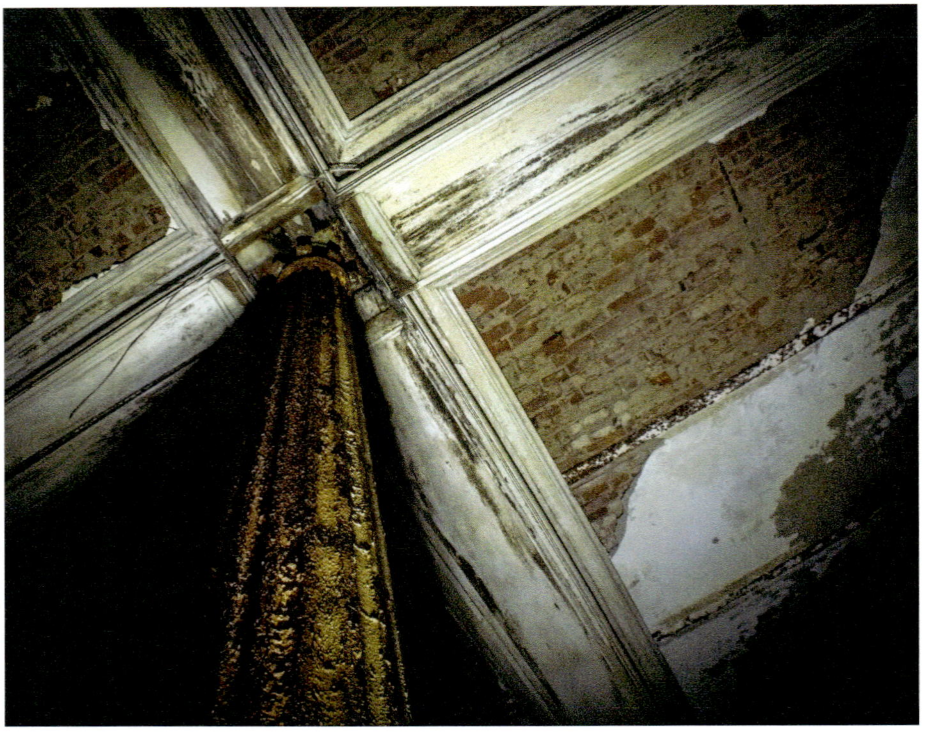

I wander the ruins at night, capturing the golden decay of the castle's support columns through the mysterious shadows. I am more downtrodden than afraid. *[Photo by Brian Cray]*

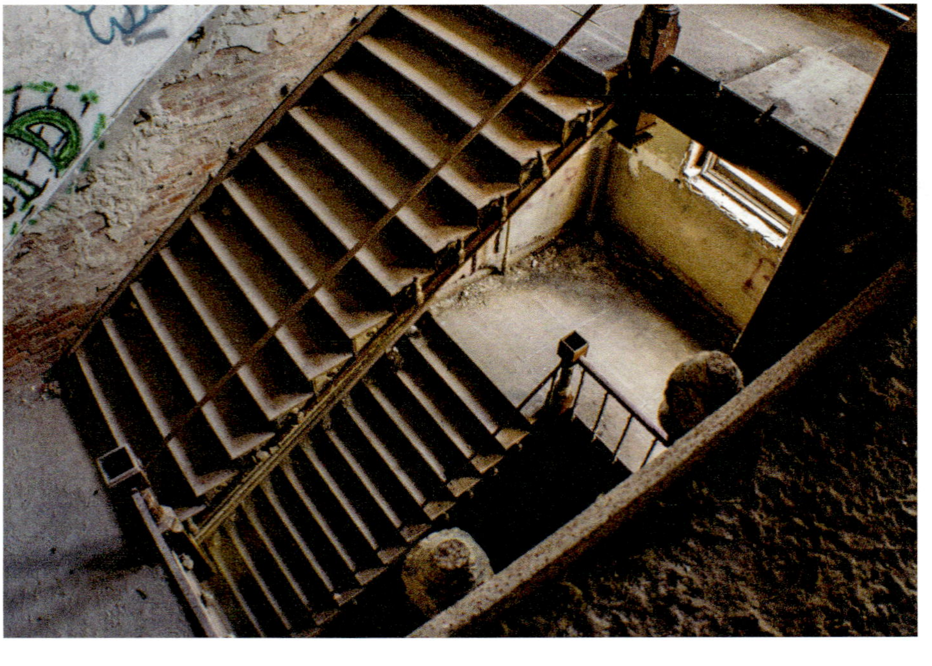

The wrought-iron balustrade wraps around the square spiral staircase blistered in rust and caked in dust shavings. *[Photo by Brian Cray]*

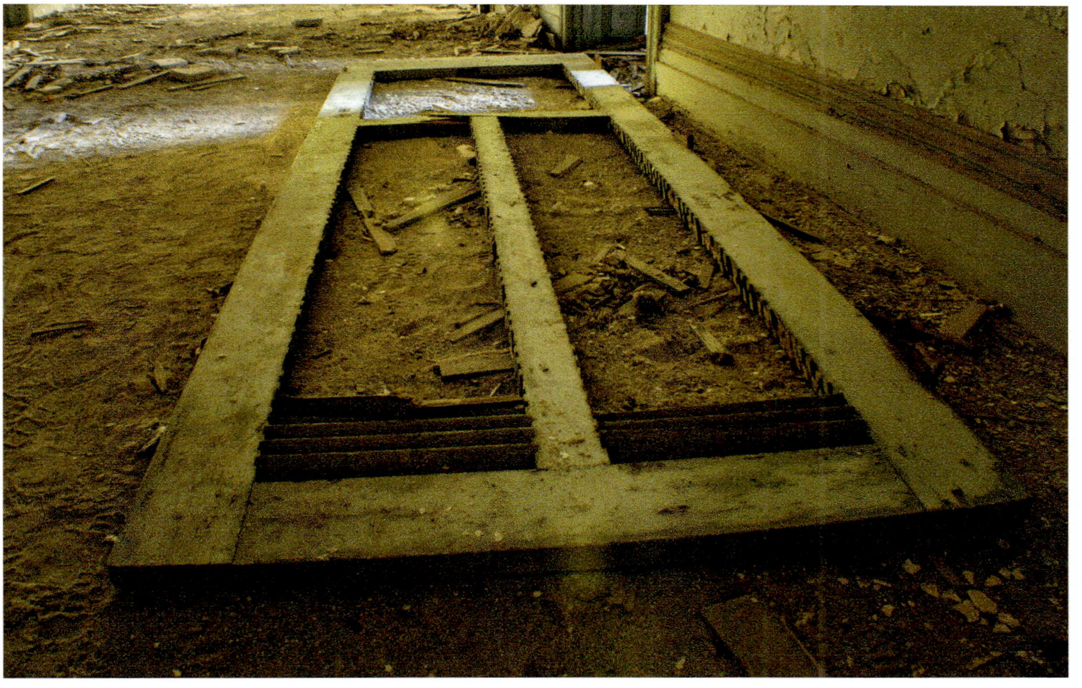

Broken doors adorn the floors as I wander the empty ruins that once held 160 patients in the new building, with another forty patients occupying the seven cottages on the hill. (Jackson, 2010) *[Photo by Brian Cray]*

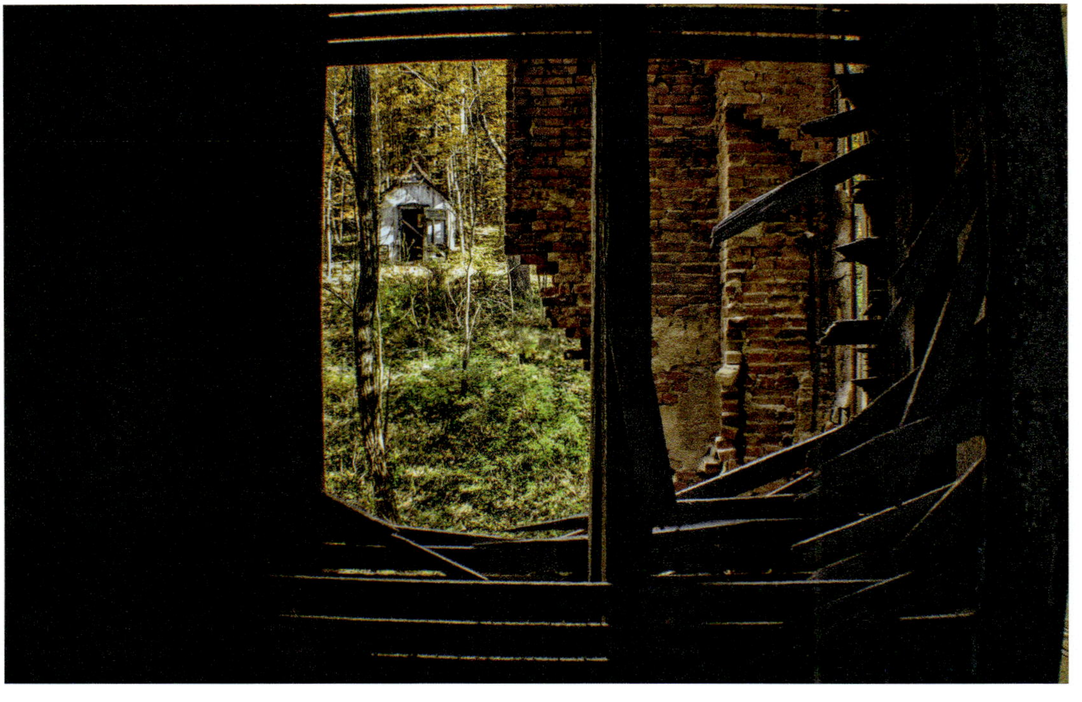

Through the dark, splintered walls shed light and muddled bricks cling to the scars of the edifice waiting like Lemmings to meet their demise. *[Photo by Brian Cray]*

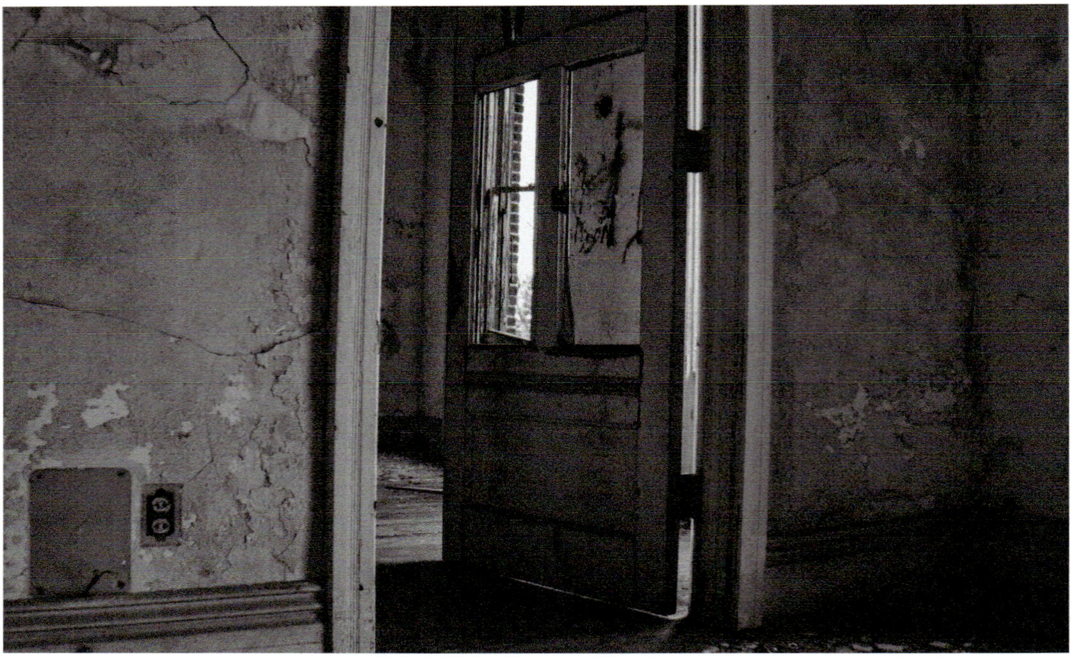

Macfadden's envision of a cult following based on his ideologies of physical fitness hit a plateau of 200 people and dwindled substantially after an affair with his secretary and an arrest in 1907 for distribution of lewd materials through the mail. (Adams, 2010) *[Photo by Brian Cray]*

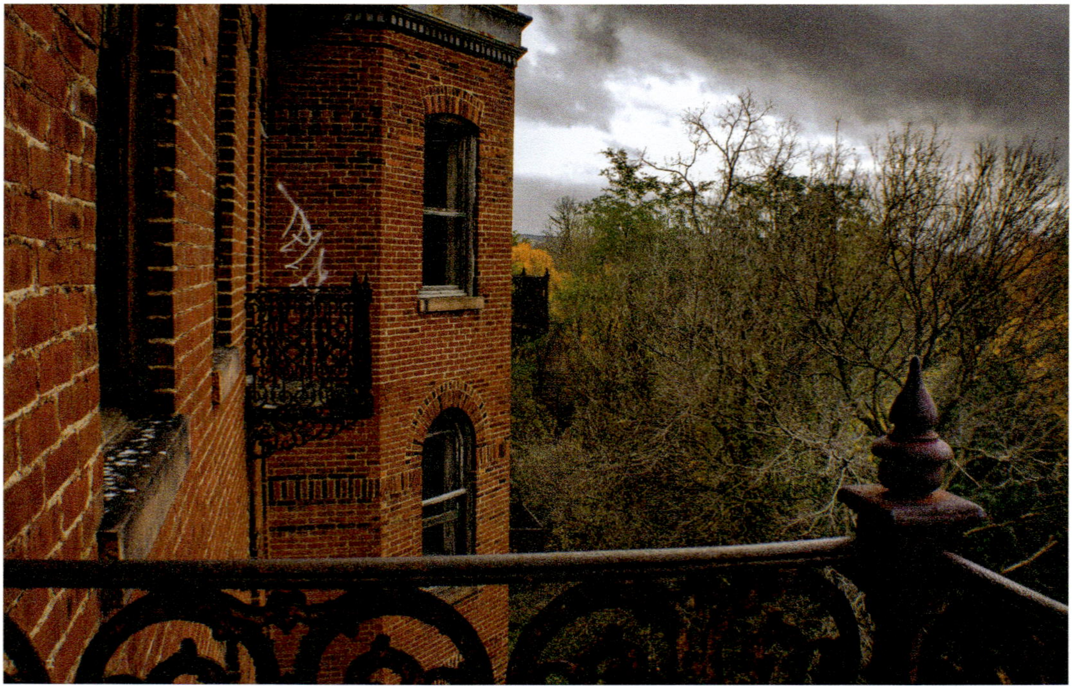

Dismal sky and barren trees add to the desolate decay on the western hillside. Don't worry I'm not standing on the balcony. *[Photo by Brian Cray]*

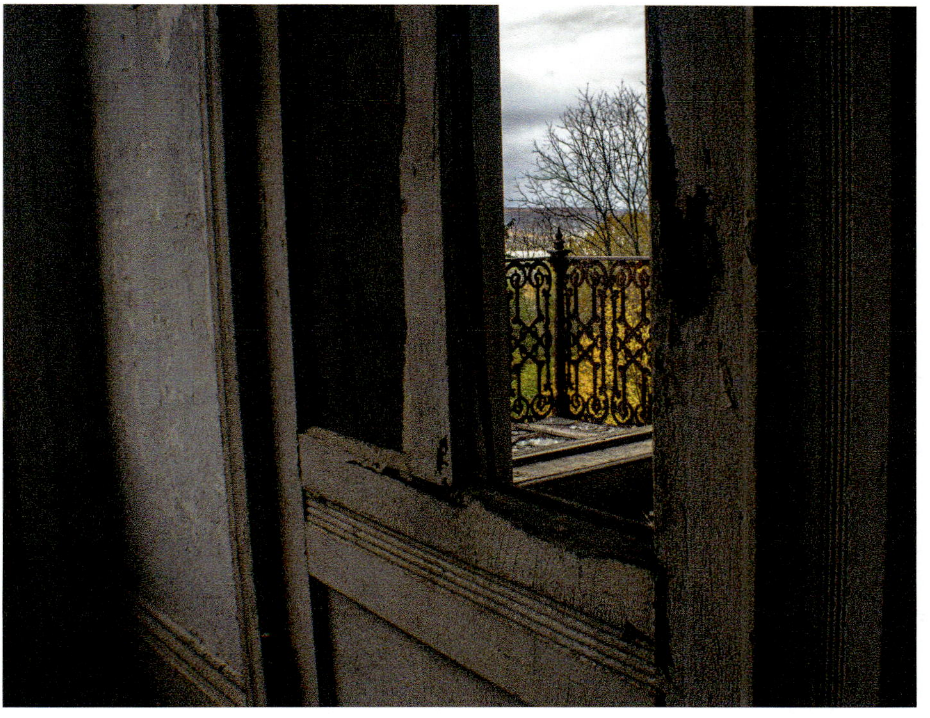

As I look out towards the balcony I wonder how an edifice with such extraordinary history, a building that pioneered the first cereal and was producing 4,000 boxes of Granula a month in its prime, is just a shell of what it once was. (Jackson, 2010) *[Photo by Brian Cray]*

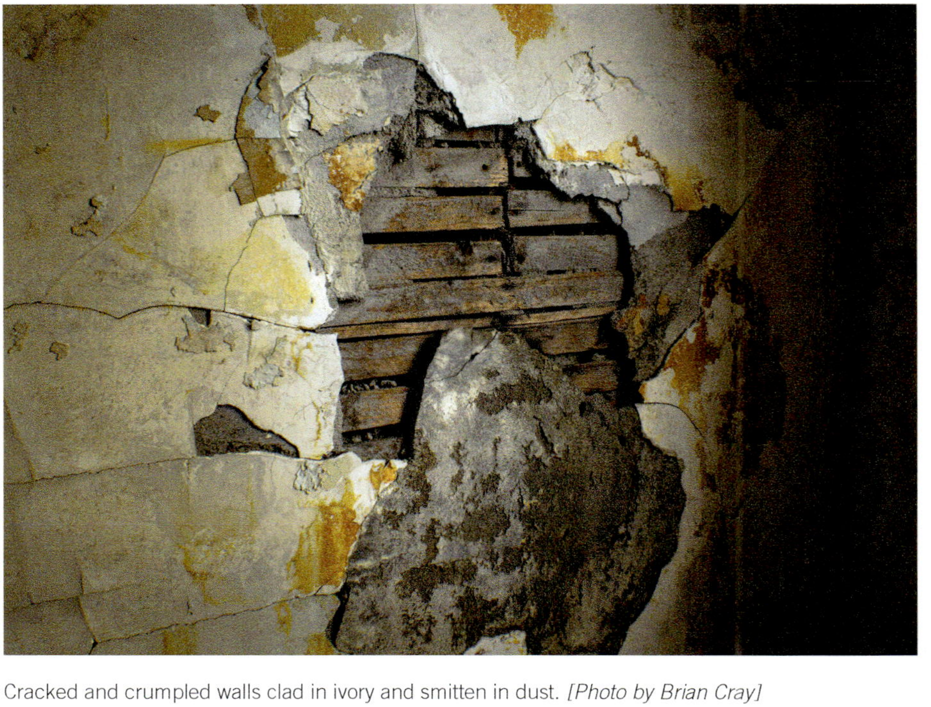

Cracked and crumpled walls clad in ivory and smitten in dust. *[Photo by Brian Cray]*

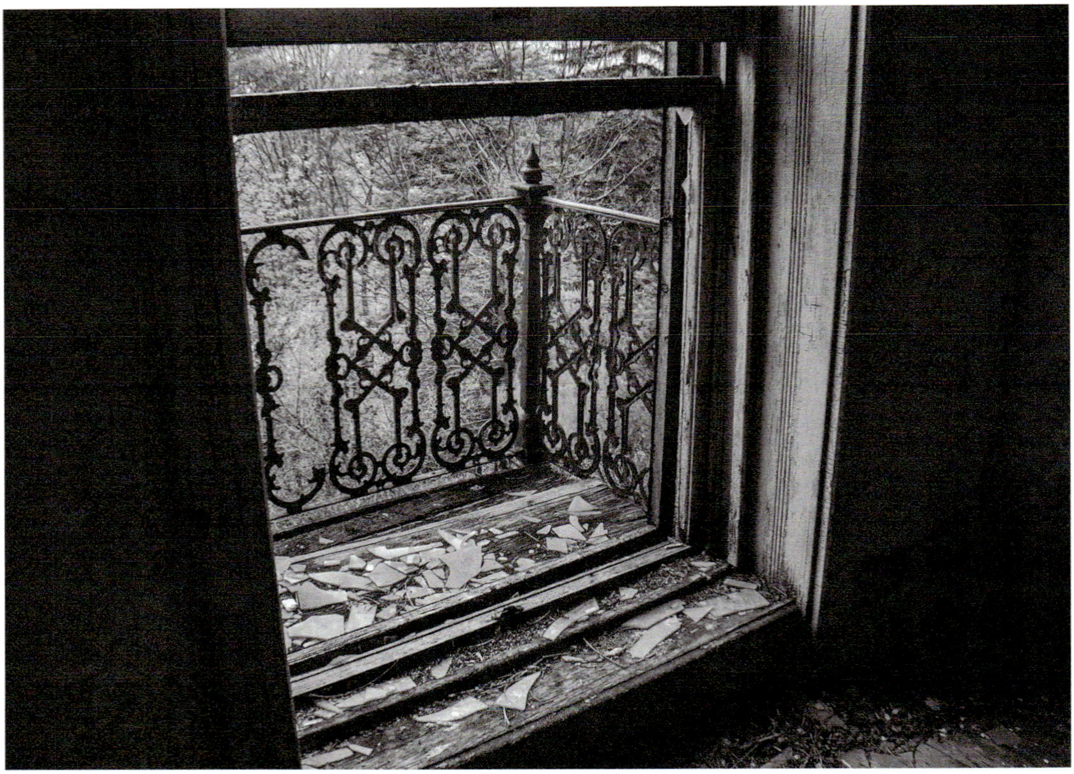

Battle Creek Sanitarium in Michigan founded by John Harvey Kellogg had more than three hundred thousand patrons pass through the institution in a span of sixty-five years. (Adams, 2010) *[Photo by Brian Cray]*

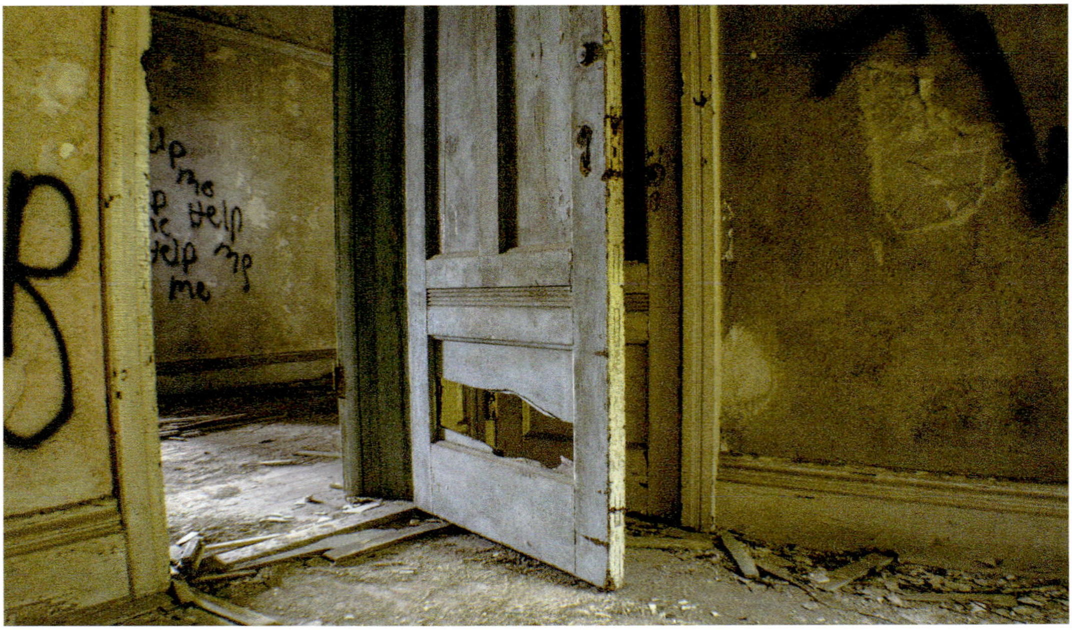

Vandalism tarnishes her insides with sub-par graffiti scribbled upon each of her empty walls. *[Photo by Brian Cray]*

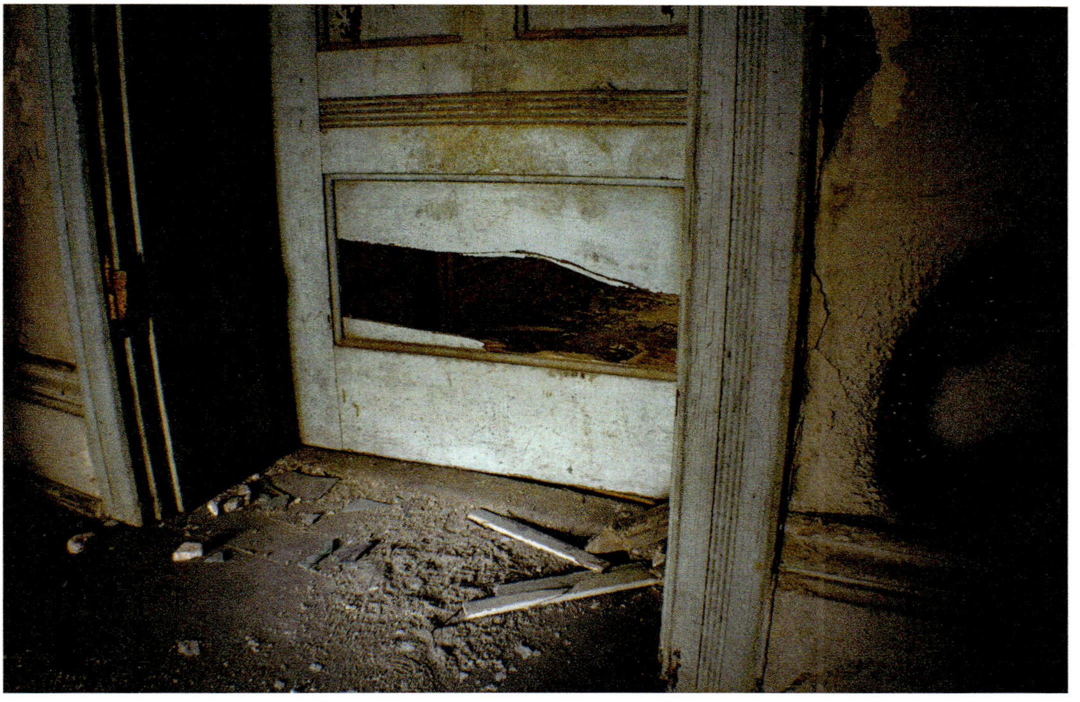

In the days of Dr. James Caleb Jackson, everyone was considered "family," but as I creep in these dark shadows, I can only feel the cries of what was left behind. *[Photo by Brian Cray]*

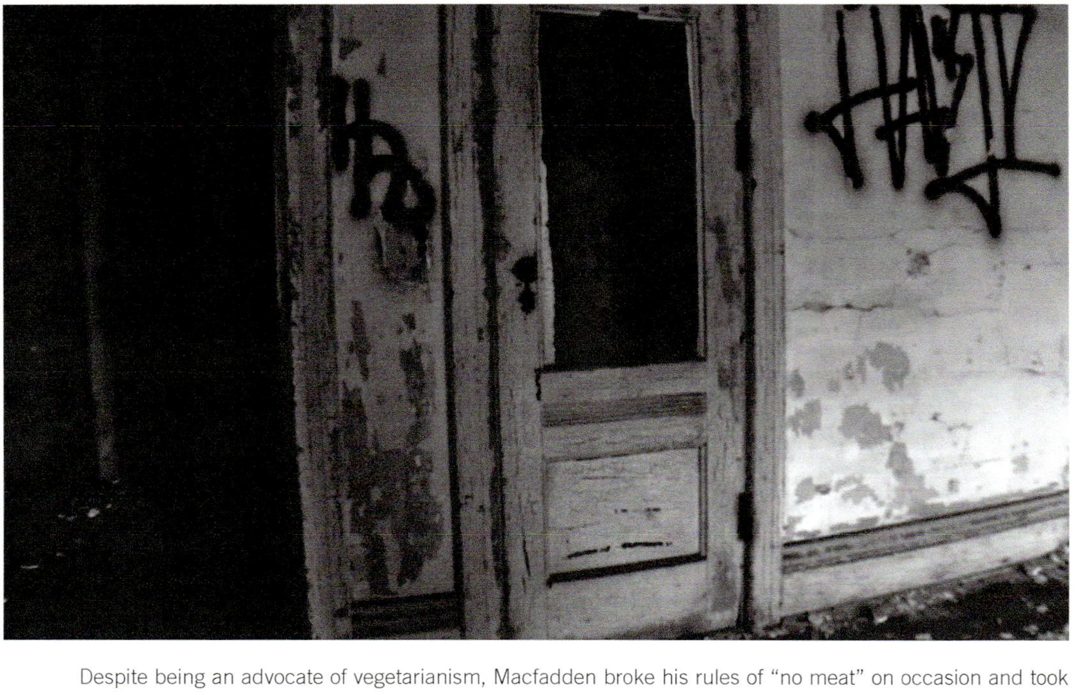

Despite being an advocate of vegetarianism, Macfadden broke his rules of "no meat" on occasion and took cheat days just like the rest of us, eating beefsteaks as rumors surfaced of a smell permeating about his room. (Adams, 2010) *[Photo by Brian Cray]*

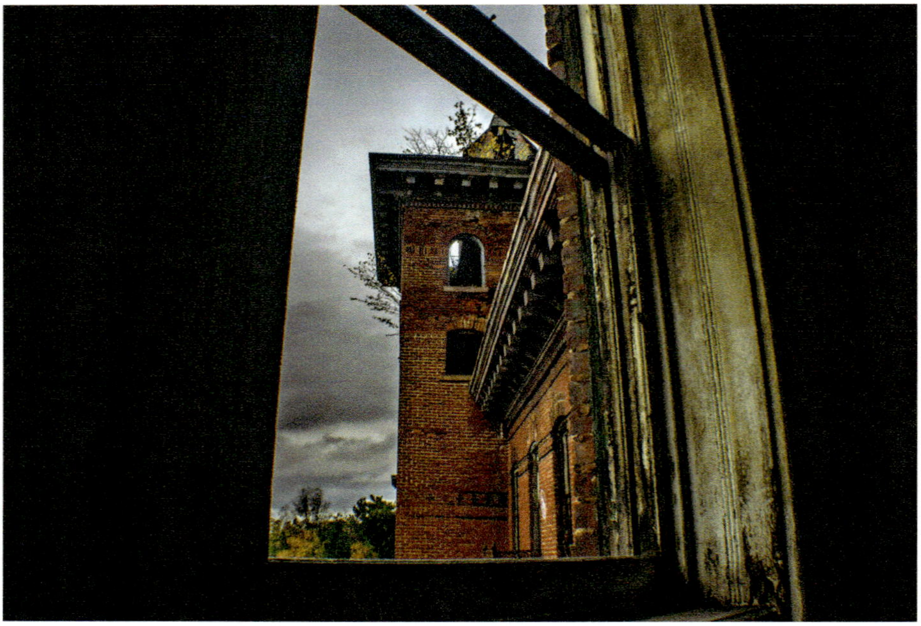

Gloomy swirls of dismal sky roll in the clouds and as I peek through a window looking at Dr. Jackson's office in the tower, I can only ponder about how he would have felt when Macfadden turned his chapel into a gymnasium. (Jackson, 2010) *[Photo by Brian Cray]*

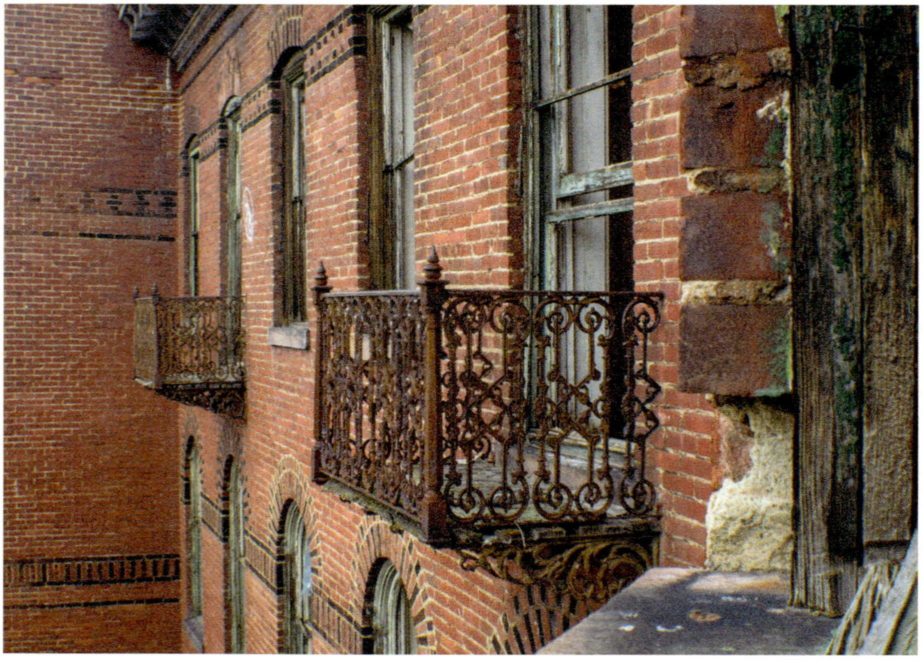

As I scrutinize the gritty wrought-iron balconies, surviving the torment of a thousand storms, I imagine what it was like to look off from her ledge 100 years ago. I imagine hearing the chickens cluck and cows moo in the nearby farm, golfers yelling "FOUR" at Brae Burns golf course and the thwack of tennis balls slicing the air by the courts. (Jackson, 2010) *[Photo by Brian Cray]*

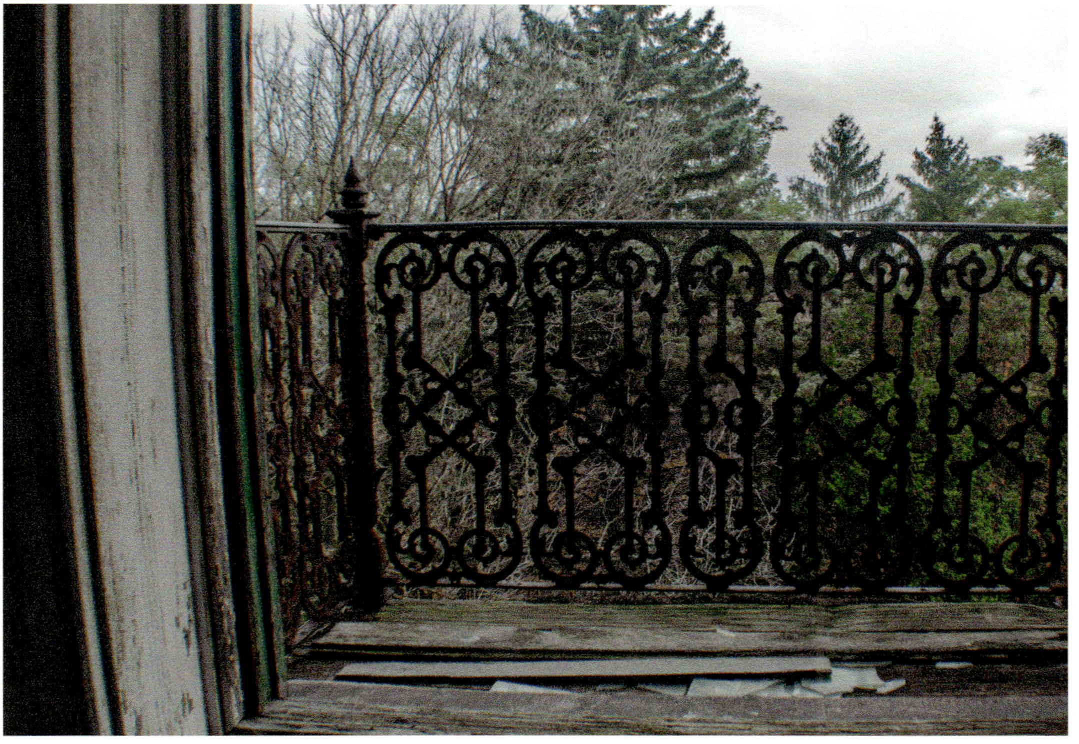

I look beyond the broken glass and splintered wood, focusing on the zigzag faces of oxidized iron crying back at me. *[Photo by Brian Cray]*

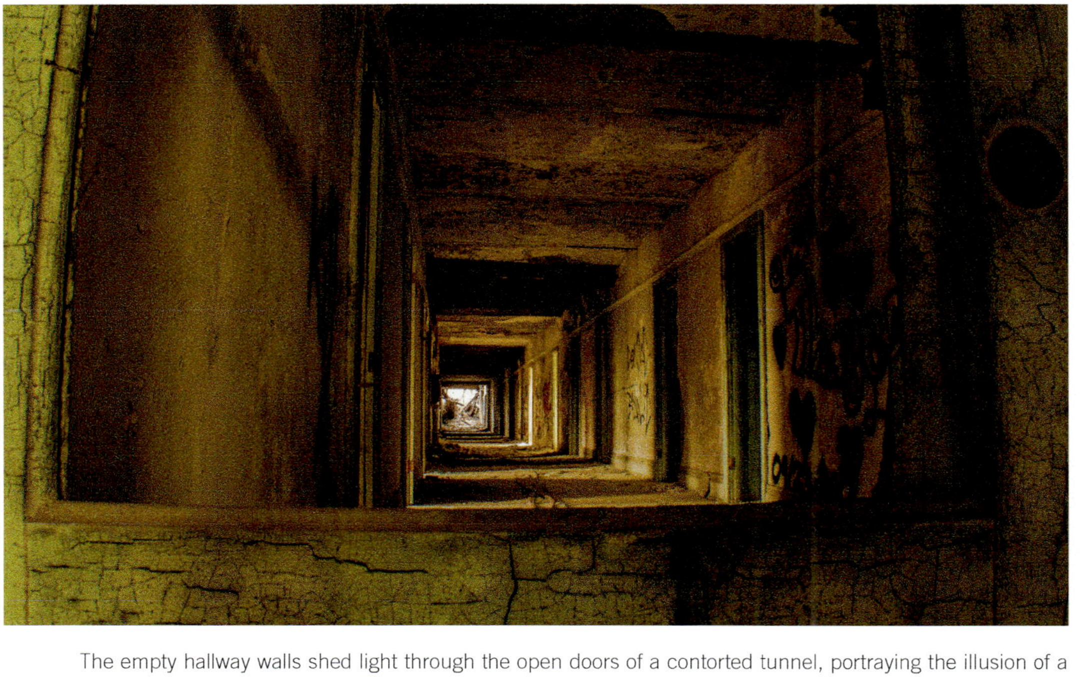

The empty hallway walls shed light through the open doors of a contorted tunnel, portraying the illusion of a tapered end. *[Photo by Brian Cray]*

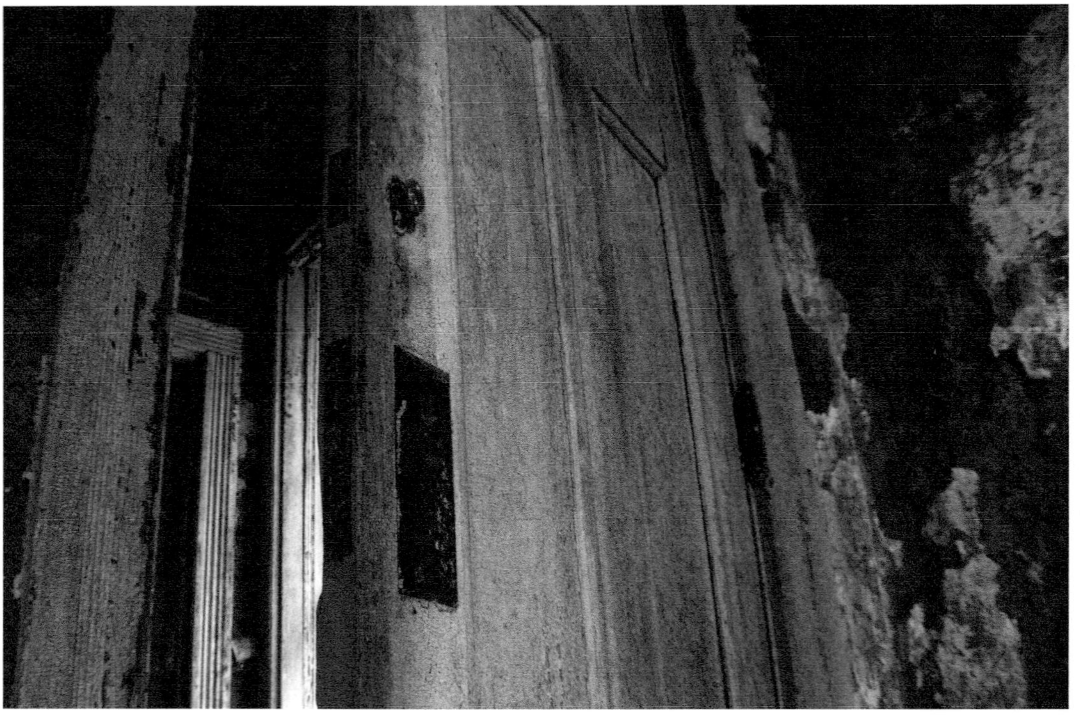

Macfadden claimed massaging the thyroid gland in men could bring back color in one's gray hair follicles. *[Photo by Brian Cray]*

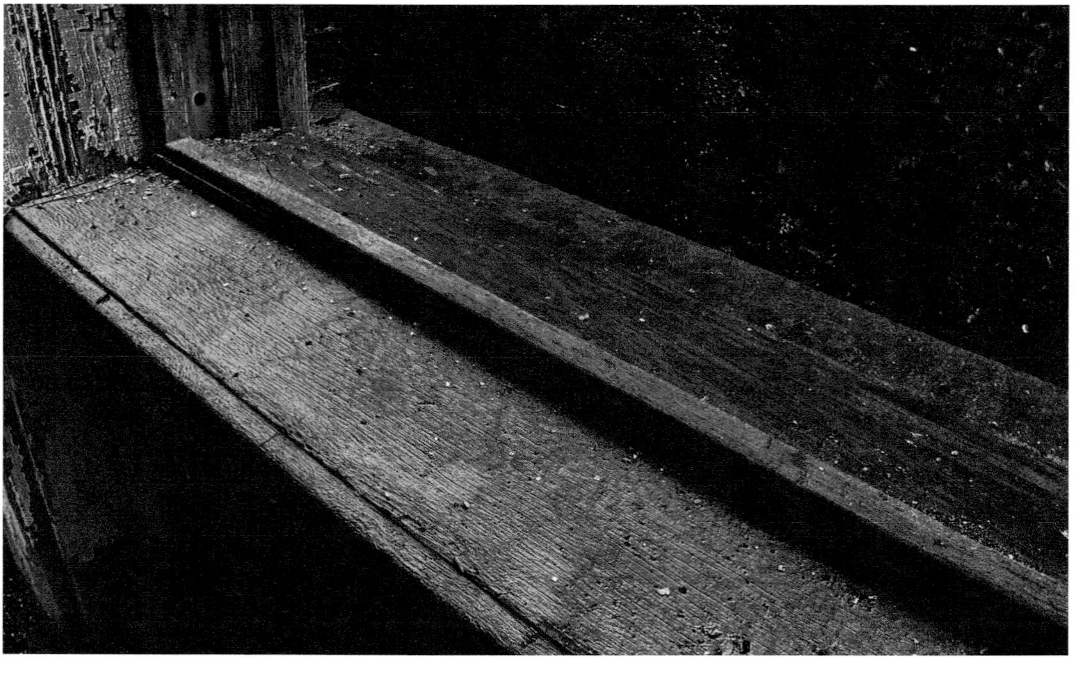

Macfadden volunteered to lead sex education programs in America to indoctrinate the youth about venereal diseases such as syphilis and gonorrhea. (Adams, 2010) *[Photo by Brian Cray]*

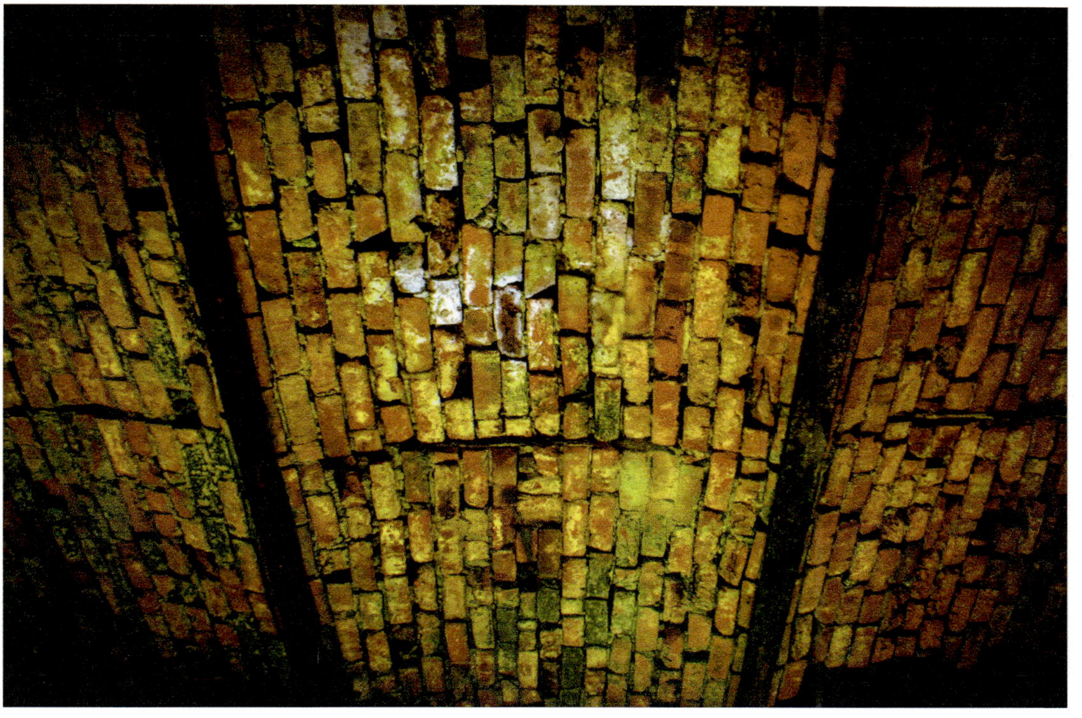

The Jack-O-Lantern ceiling of brick lines the walls and the halls of the castle, making it "fireproof" after its reconstruction in 1883, which is how they "sold" it to patrons! *[Photo by Brian Cray]*

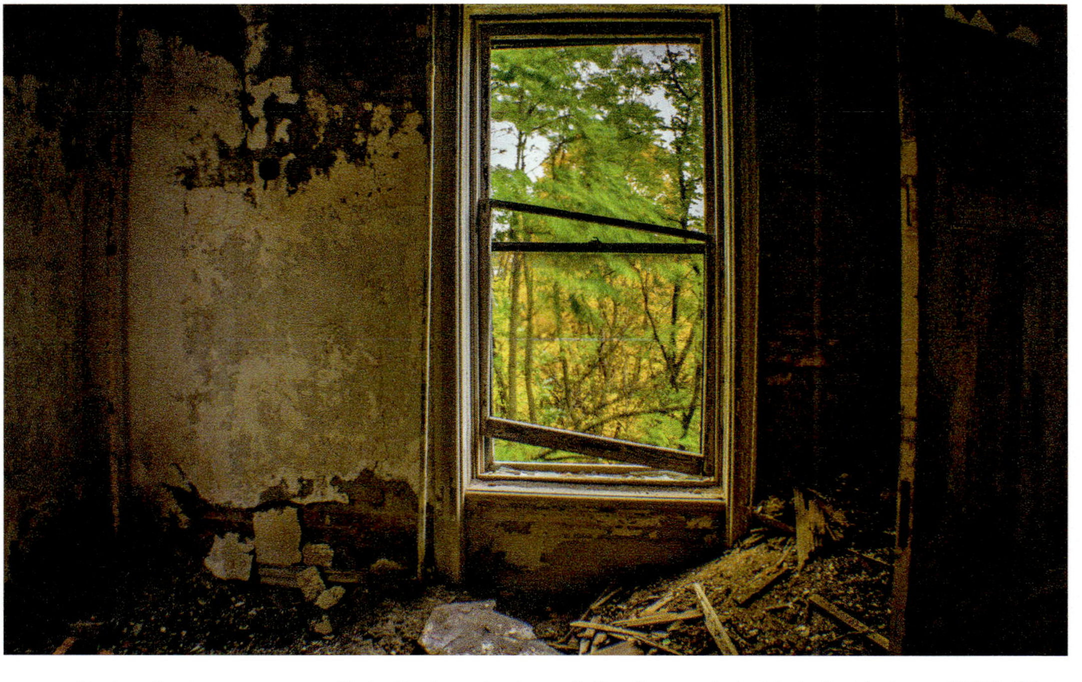

Each patient room was supplied with steam heat, ventilating flues and electric bells. (Jackson, 2010) *[Photo by Brian Cray]*

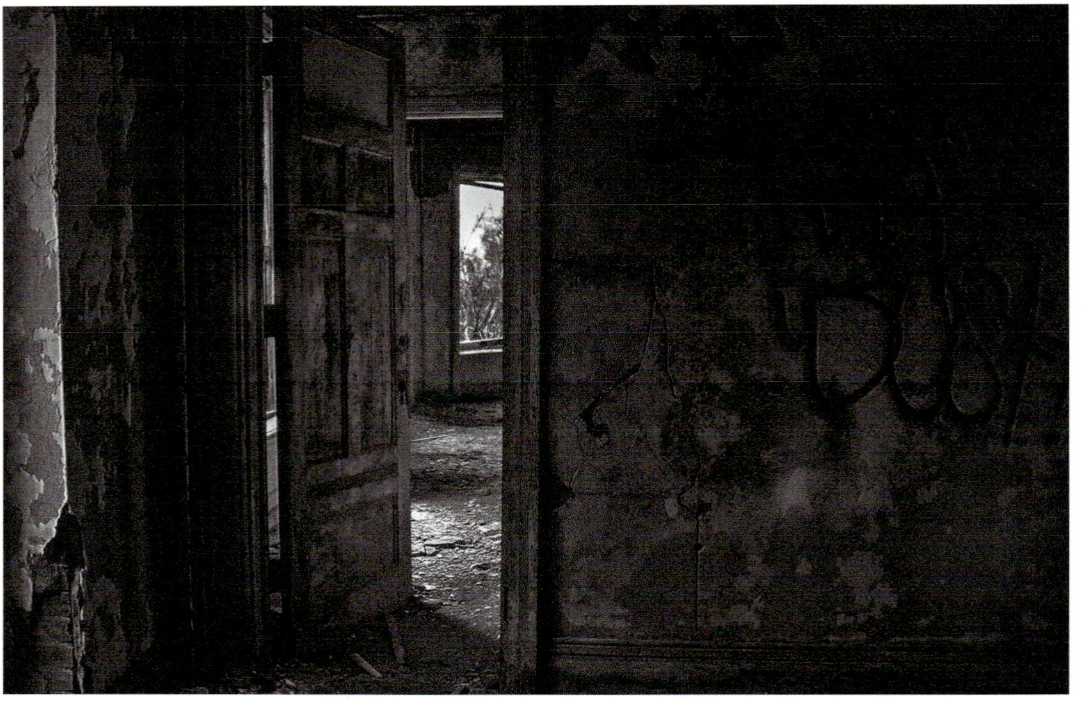

Macfadden also wrote of political topics in his magazine titled *Macfadden's Weekly, The Cry for Justice, and Fair Play*, where he spoke of the hindrance of monopolies, the importance of great public education and how the working men and women of this country need rights. (Adams, 2010) *[Photo by Brian Cray]*

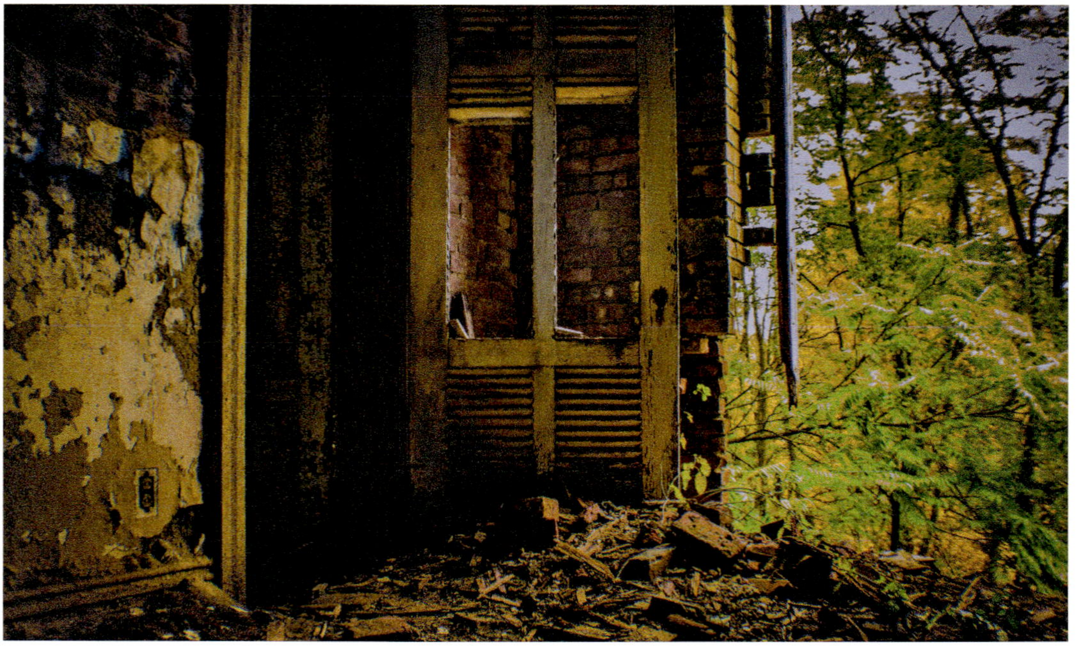

It's dark. It's eerie. I fear falling through her open wounds waiting for bricks to plunge to the ground like Lemmings with a canvas of deep green forest thriving beyond her dying walls. *[Photo by Brian Cray]*

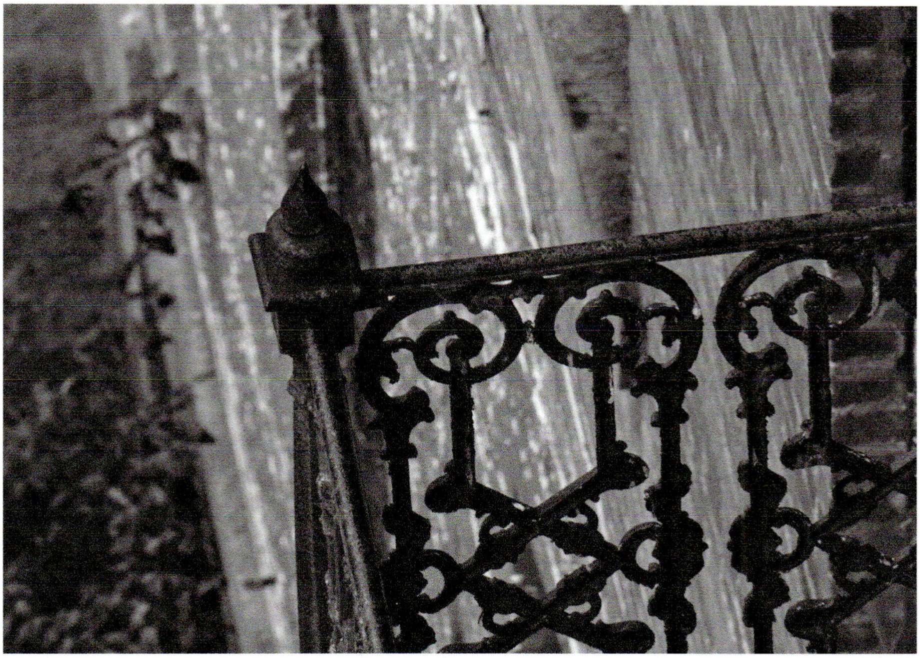

In all the years the *Physical Culture* magazine delivered witty content to its subscribers, it never covered any topics practiced by "real" licensed medical doctors. (Adams, 2010) *[Photo by Brian Cray]*

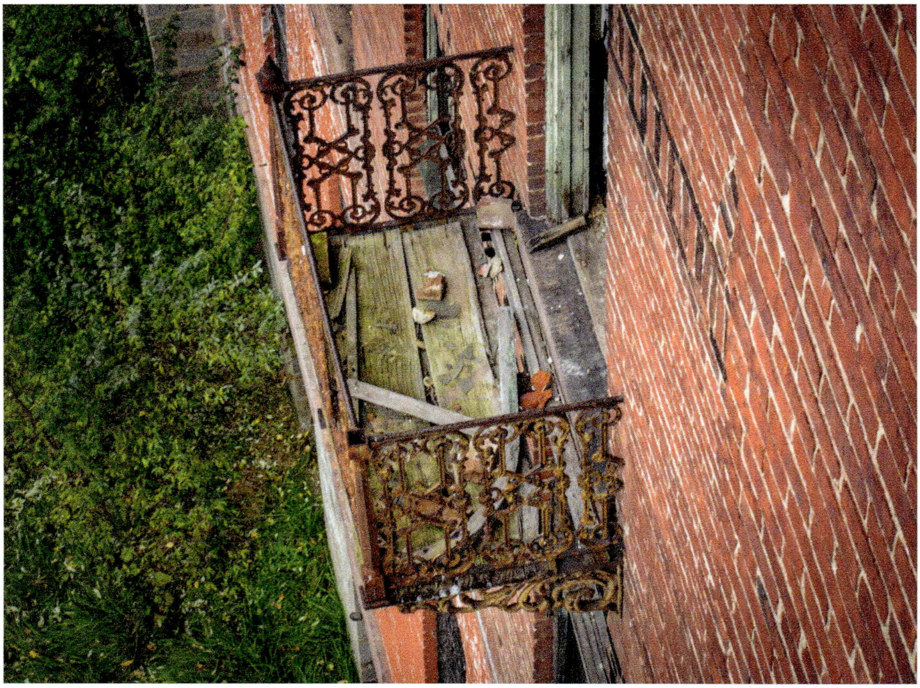

Fresh flowers adorned the Chapel and the corridors of the San, so it's no wonder their balconies marveled in sophistication. I bet when the Brightside Library opened in 1891, many patrons read amongst the balconies looking out at the endless beauty along the hillside. *[Photo by Brian Cray]*

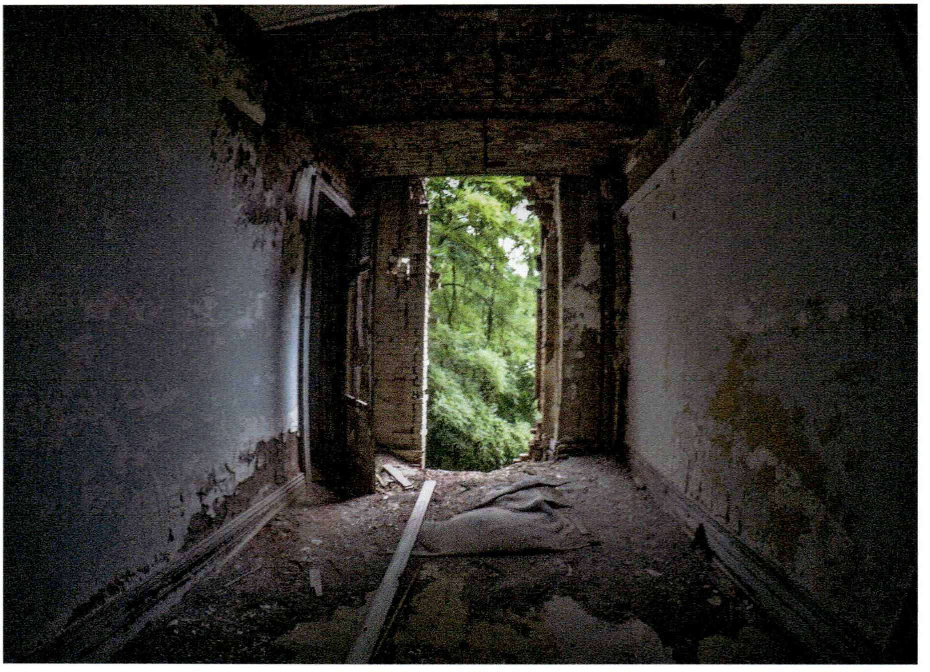

The door to this private room leads to nowhere but a painful plunge to the ground floor. If you live you won't experience water shock treatment or hydrotherapy like the patients of "Our Home on the Hillside." *[Photo by Brian Cray]*

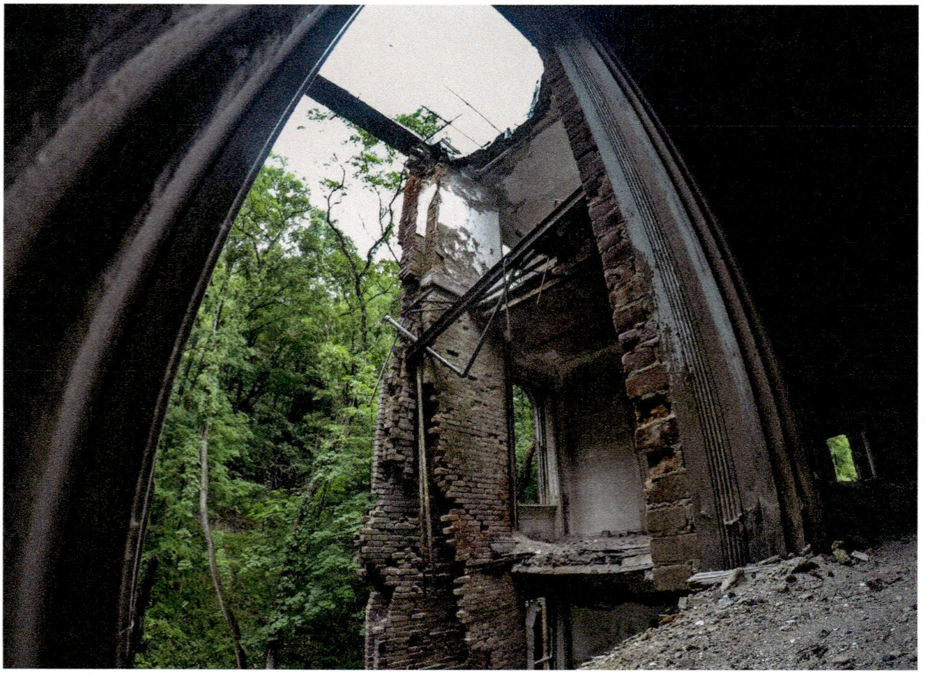

Brick-by-brick she fades away with the abyss of deep green forest as her scars widen from the vice of Mother Nature's grip. *[Photo by Brian Cray]*

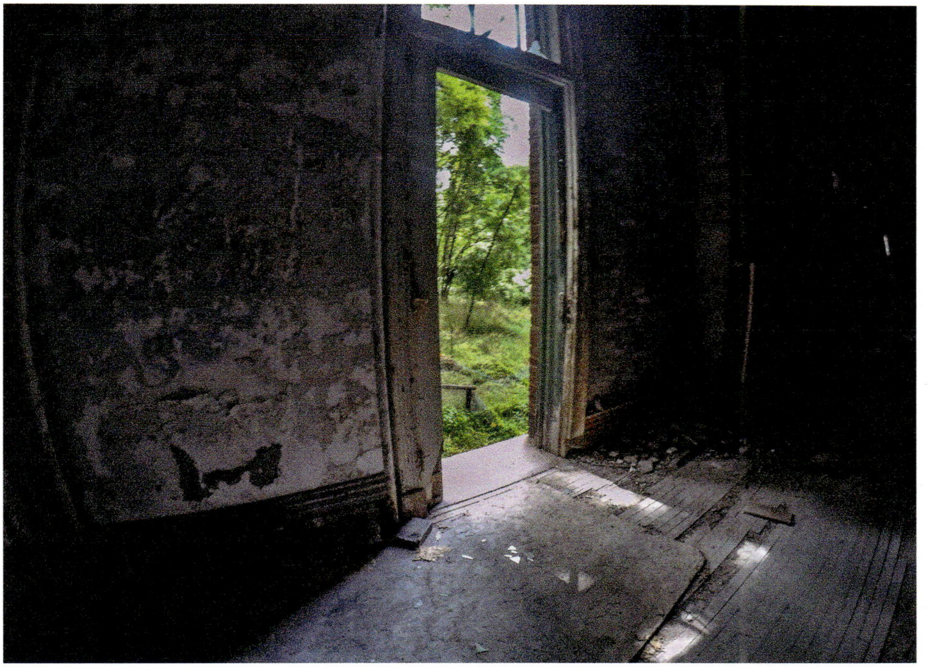

Here I stand looking out one of windowless panes while watching my steps on the creaky floorboards. Dust, dirt, and rubble only piled up as I continued my trek deeper into the castle of forgotten history. *[Photo by Brian Cray]*

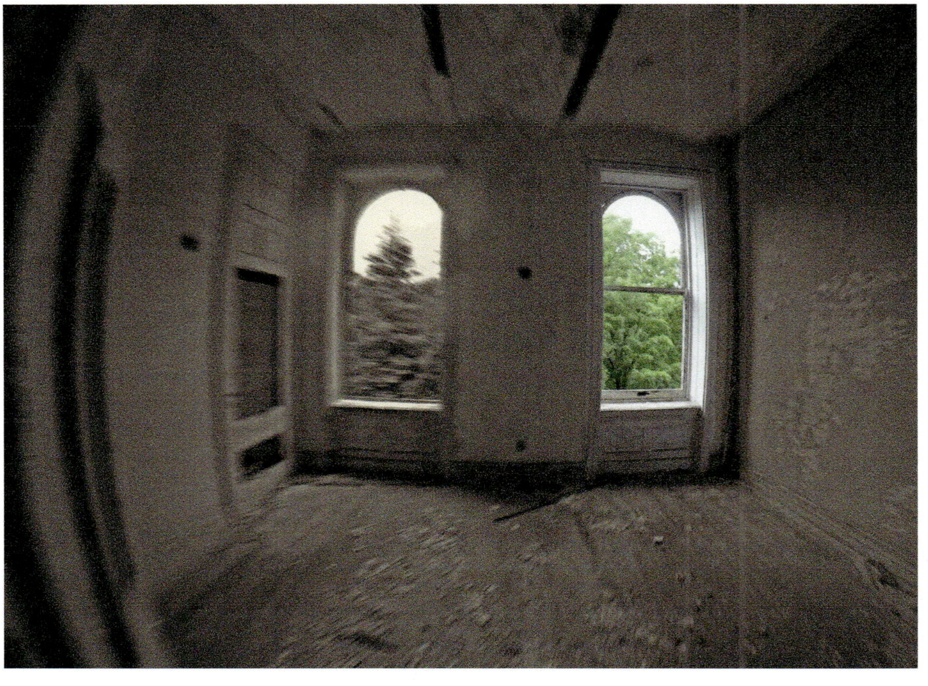

Keep both eyes open as you wander her barren rooms and explore her loose floors so you don't become a distant memory like her past. *[Photo by Brian Cray]*

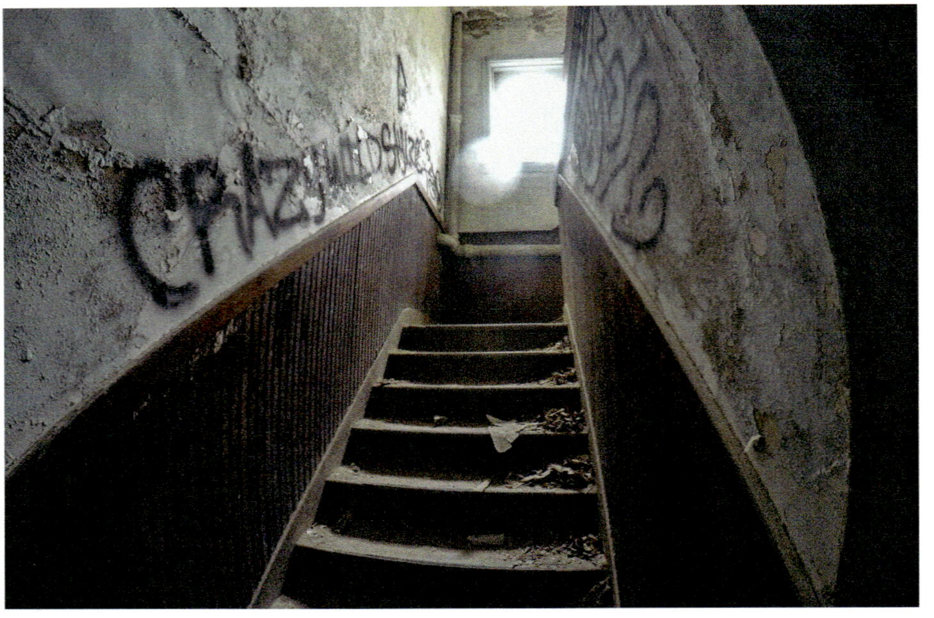

I wander up the last flight of stairs before turning the corner to explore the ruins left behind on the rooftop. For some reason I feel like dancing. Maybe it's the view overlooking the town of Dansville or the thought of lavish rooftop parties from the Physical Culture Hotel. *[Photo by Brian Cray]*

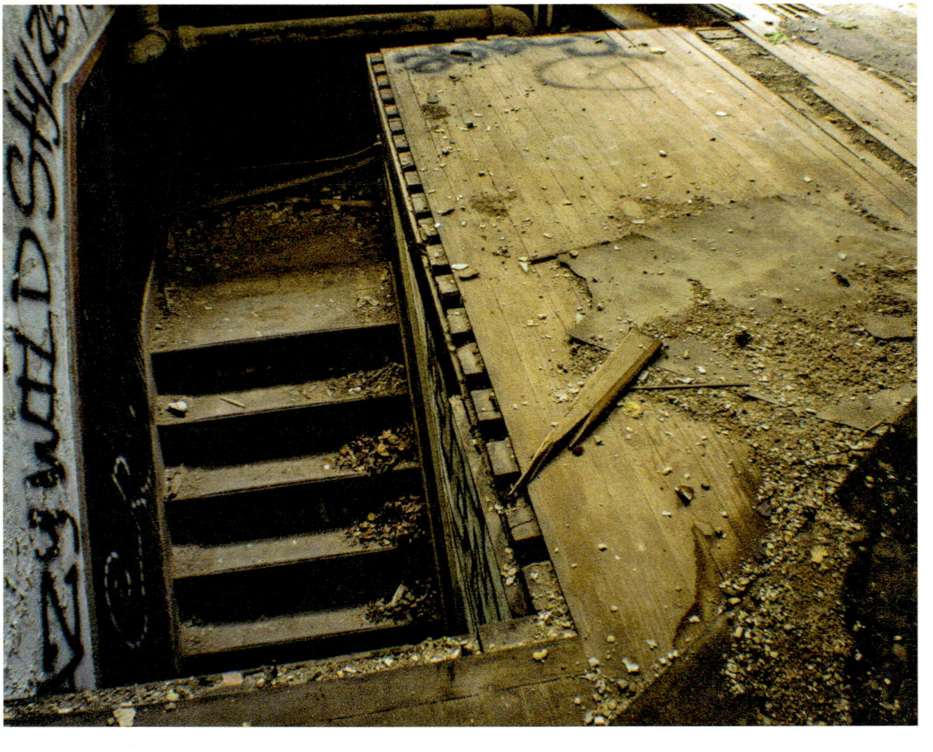

I stop under the creaking of loose, splintered, wood panels, avoiding the pits leading to the floor below. *[Photo by Brian Cray]*

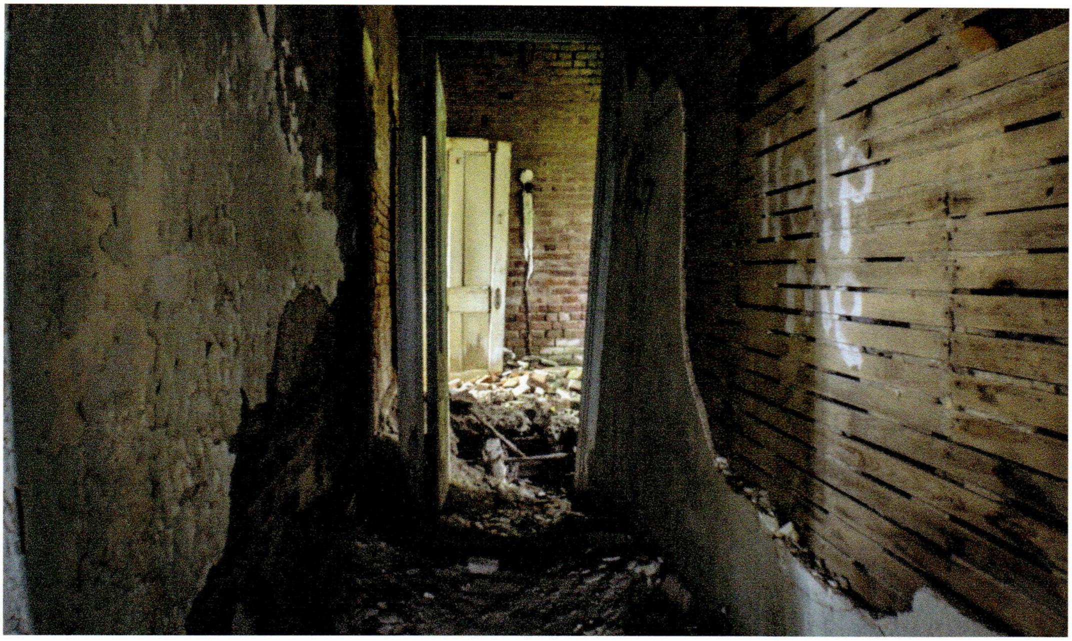

Sunken floors and bare walls suffer from years of brutal weather making these "club rooms" inaccessible to explore. *[Photo by Brian Cray]*

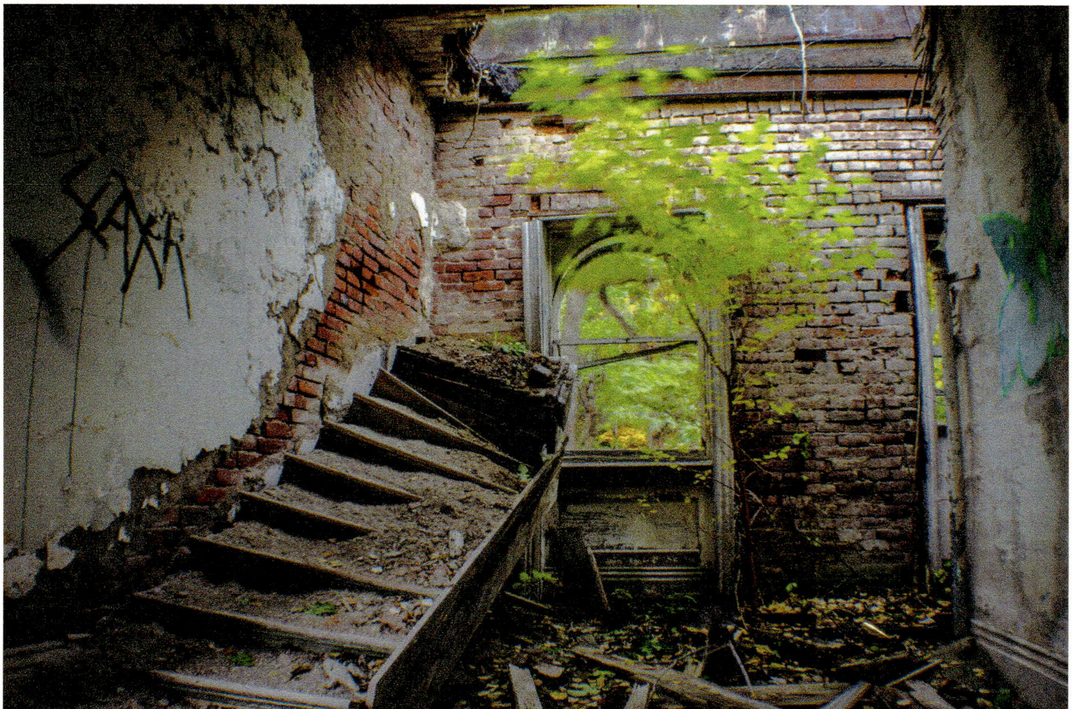

Looking towards the window, I wonder if the trees calmed them, the way they calm me as I stand in this eerie quiet shell of what once birthed hope and joy to so many. *[Photo by Brian Cray]*

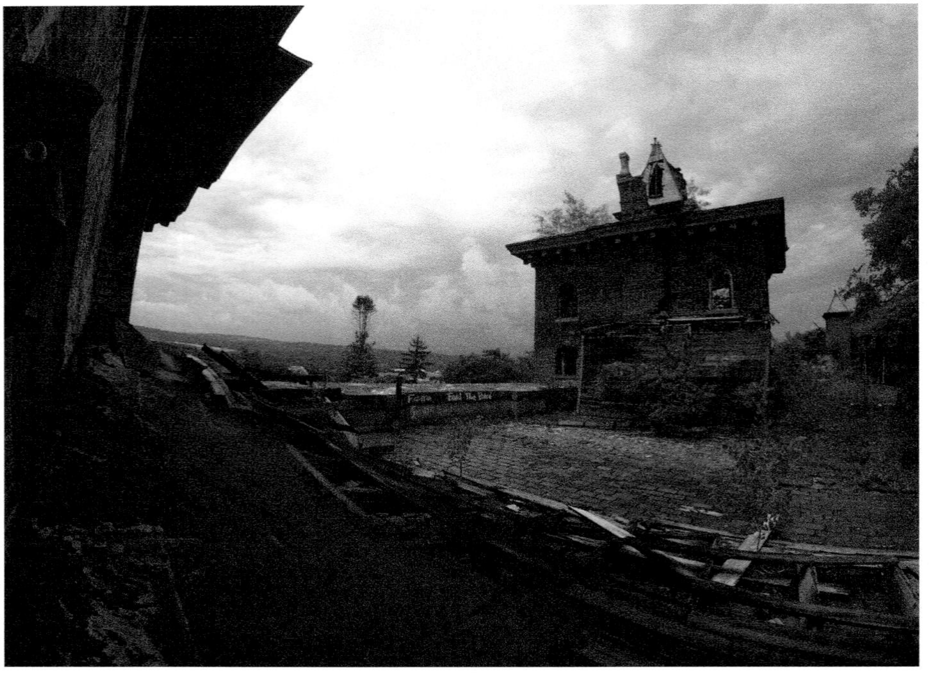

As I stare off at the trees flowering amongst the brittle bricks of the decaying rooftop, my mind wanders. I imagine groups of people dirty dancing, laughing, and gossiping over which celebrities have visited the P.C., with that one man sneaking drinks out of his flask because no one parties without alcohol, even in the 1900s. *[Photo by Brian Cray]*

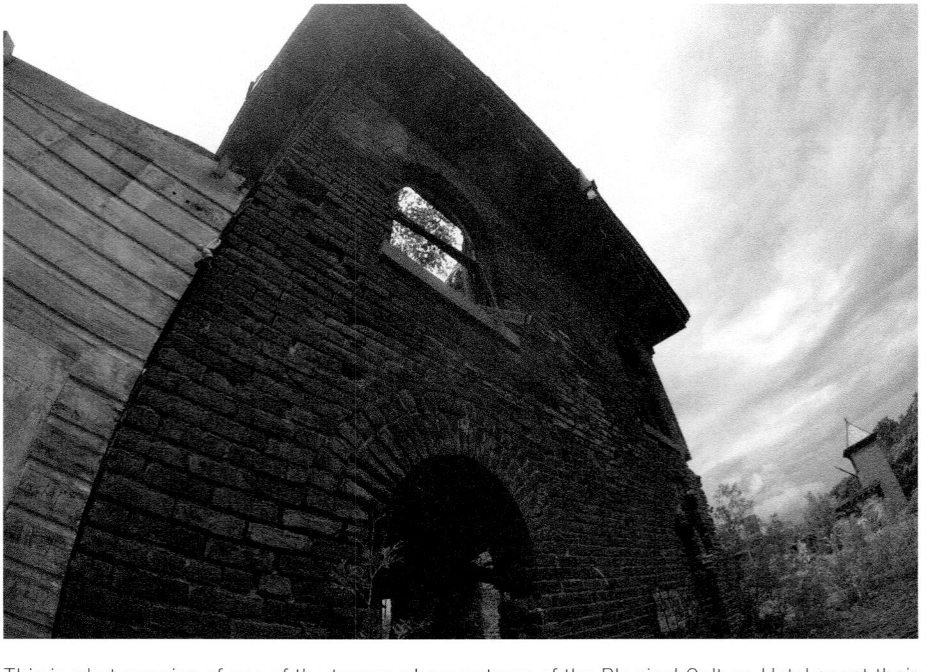

This is what remains of one of the towers where patrons of the Physical Culture Hotel spent their afternoons sunbathing amidst the rooftop. *[Photo by Brian Cray]*

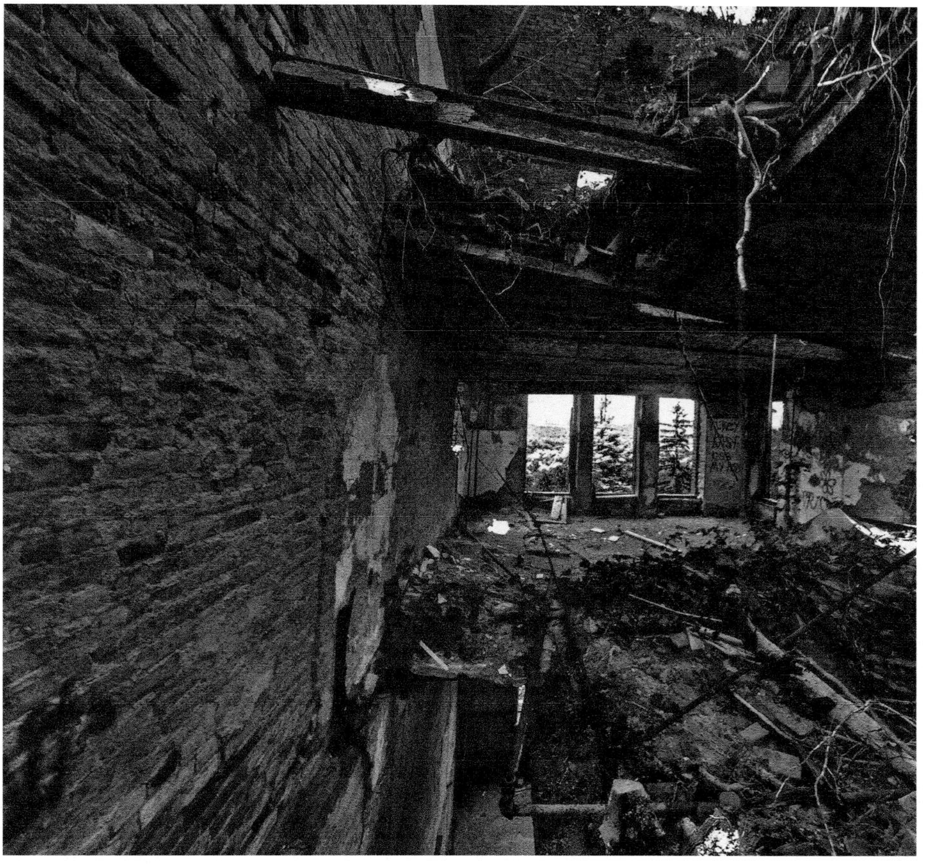

The second floor to the tower slumps at her supports as I look through the eyes of paneless windows, wondering what Dr. James Caleb Jackson's office looked like years ago. *[Photo by Brian Cray]*

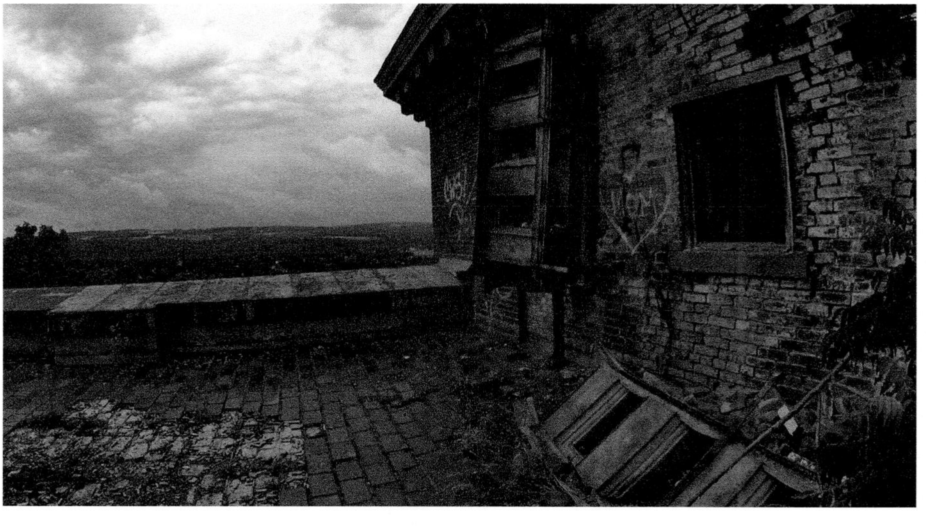

The mangled metal along the rooftop scattered among crackled bits of brick and grout die with the rest of her walls. *[Photo by Brian Cray]*

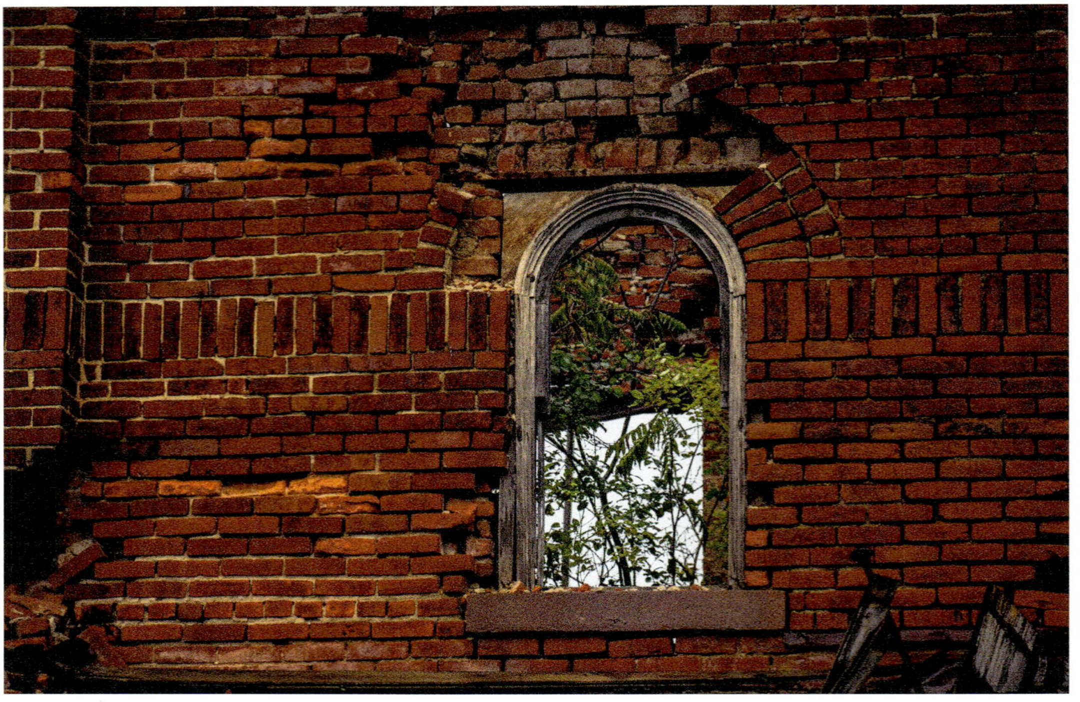

Through this window of the tower on the sixth floor over the entrance of the sanatorium was Dr. James Caleb Jackson's office. (Jackson, 2010) *[Photo by Brian Cray]*

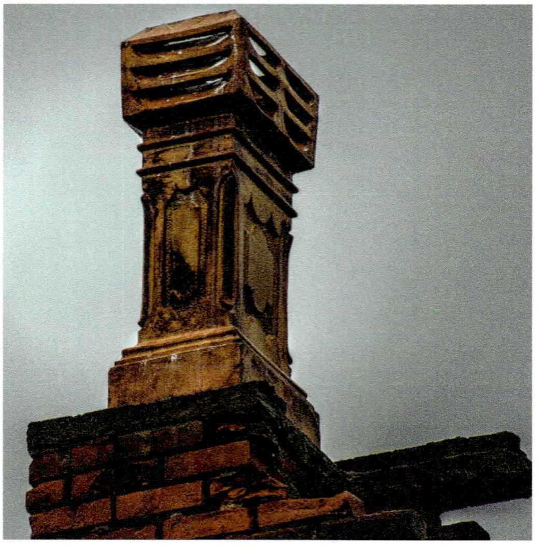

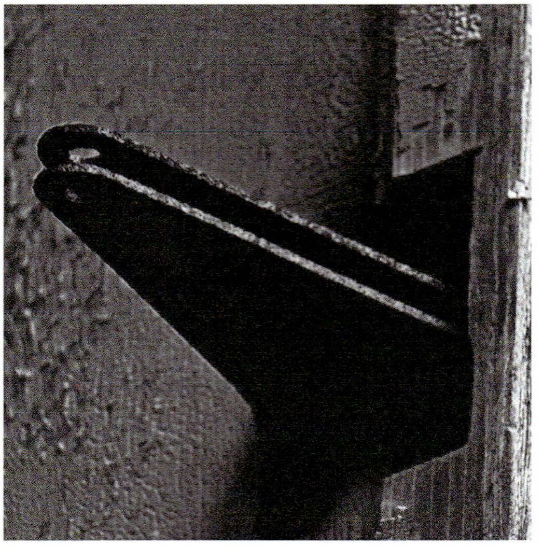

Above left: As I look out through a "club room" I can see the oxidized remnants smudged along an old chimney. These rooms cost $10 a week per person, while other rooms went as high as $30. (Jackson, 2010) *[Photo by Brian Cray]*

Above right: Upton Sinclair wrote occasional columns in Macfadden's *Physical Culture* magazine and also vacationed at his sanatorium in Battle Creek where he enjoyed fasting and the milk diet. (Adams, 2010) *[Photo by Brian Cray]*

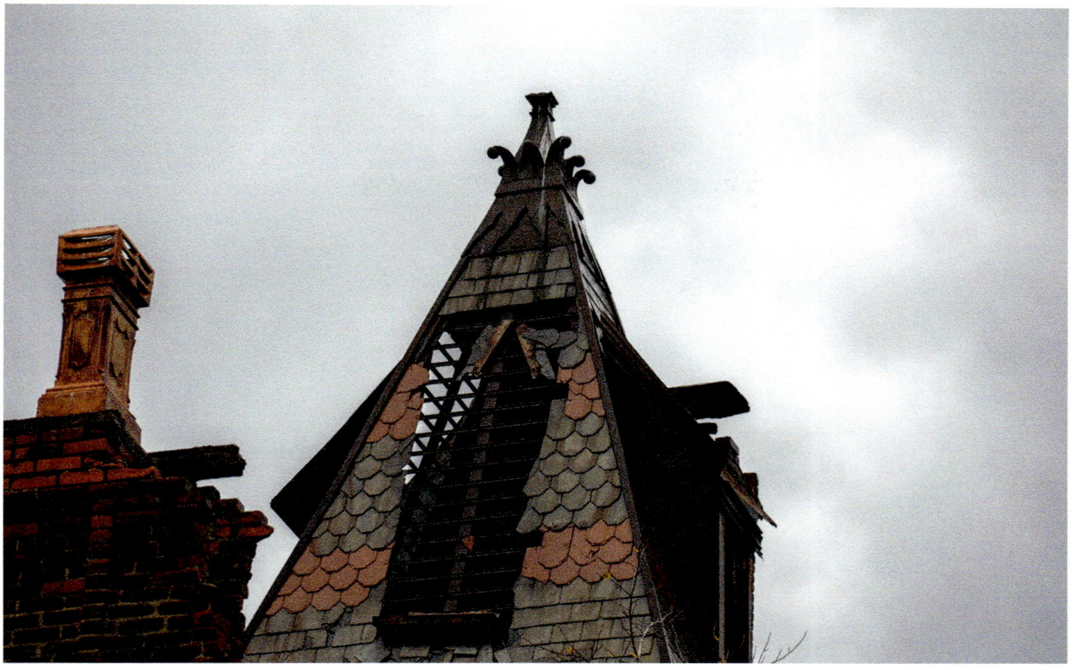

The steeple above Dr. Jackson's office wastes away with time as panels deteriorate and open up to the ferocity of seasons. *[Photo by Brian Cray]*

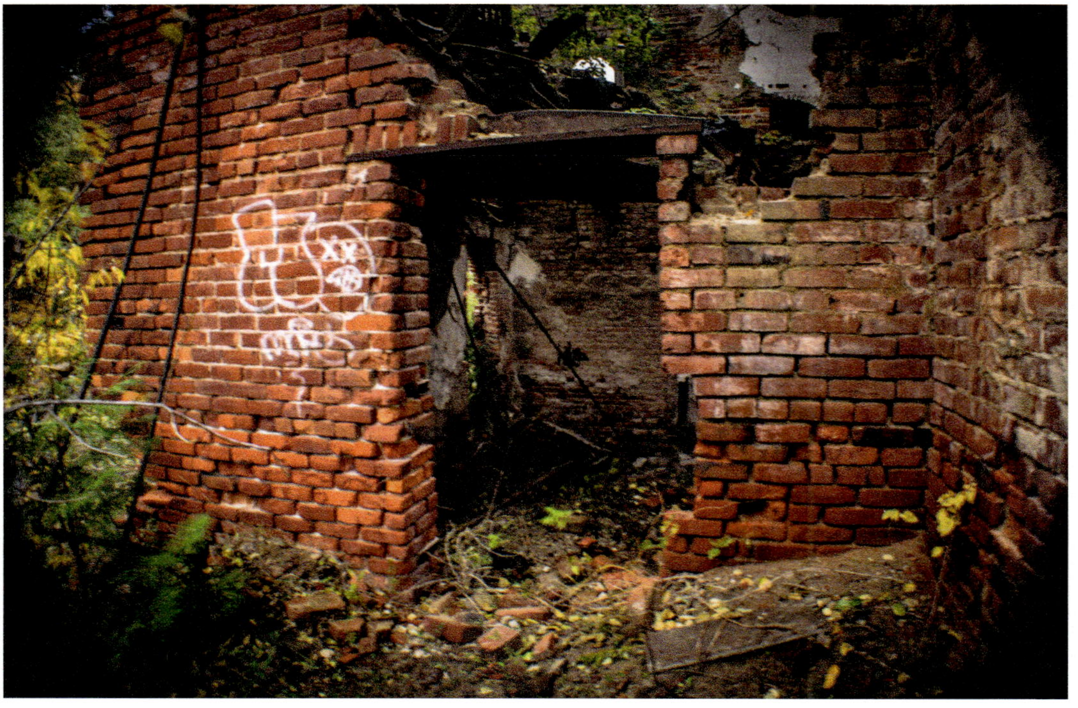

Weathered bricks wash away before my eyes and with each loose brick and drooping joist, she loses her strength to stand. Soon her distressed reds will bear the same fate as Dr. Jackson's. *[Photo by Brian Cray]*

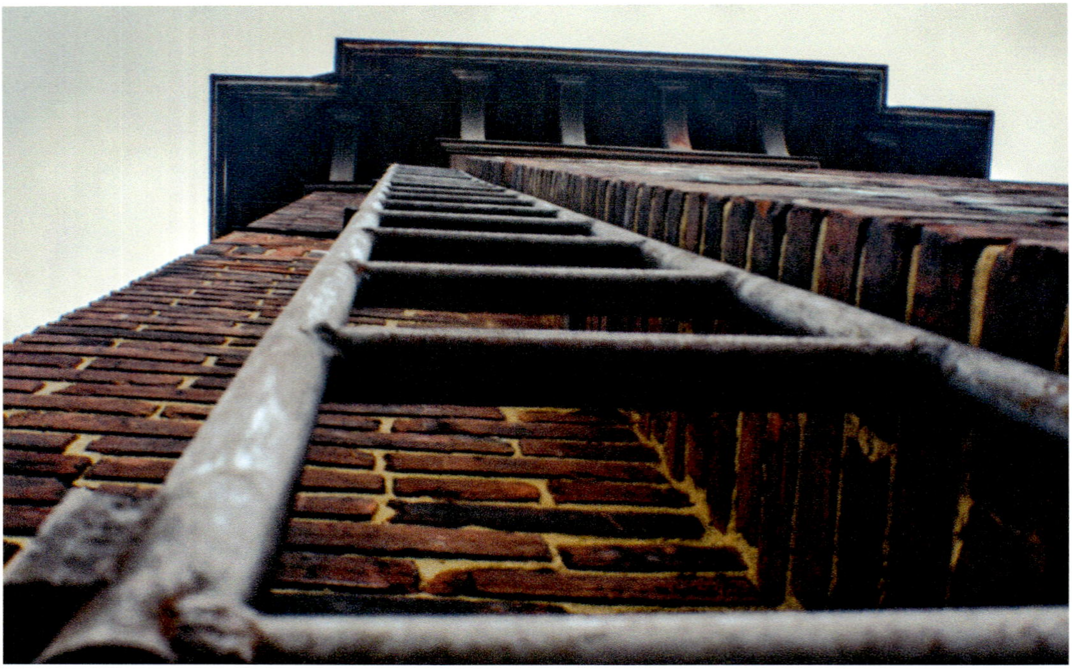

A climb to the top of Dr. Jackson's office looks harmless from this angle, but I will only take so many risks and her wounds are too deep. *[Photo by Brian Cray]*

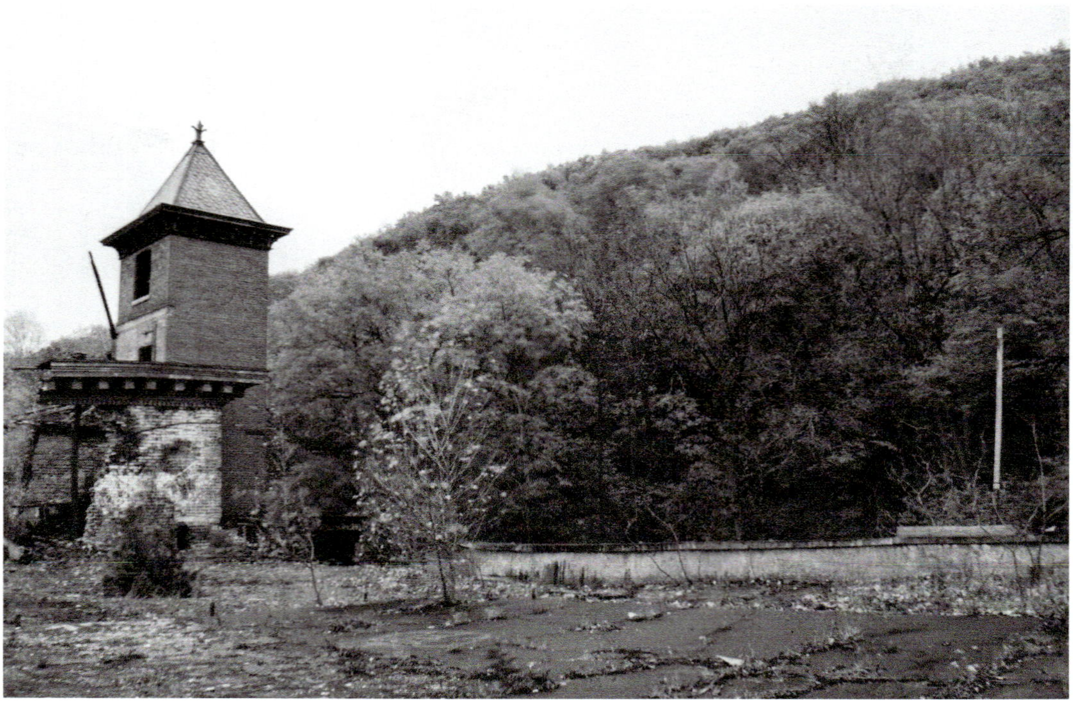

Macfadden truly believed that the practices of physcultopathy garnered near immunity to germs and through healthy diet and living one could clear their body of impurities and all disease. (Adams, 2010) *[Photo by Brian Cray]*

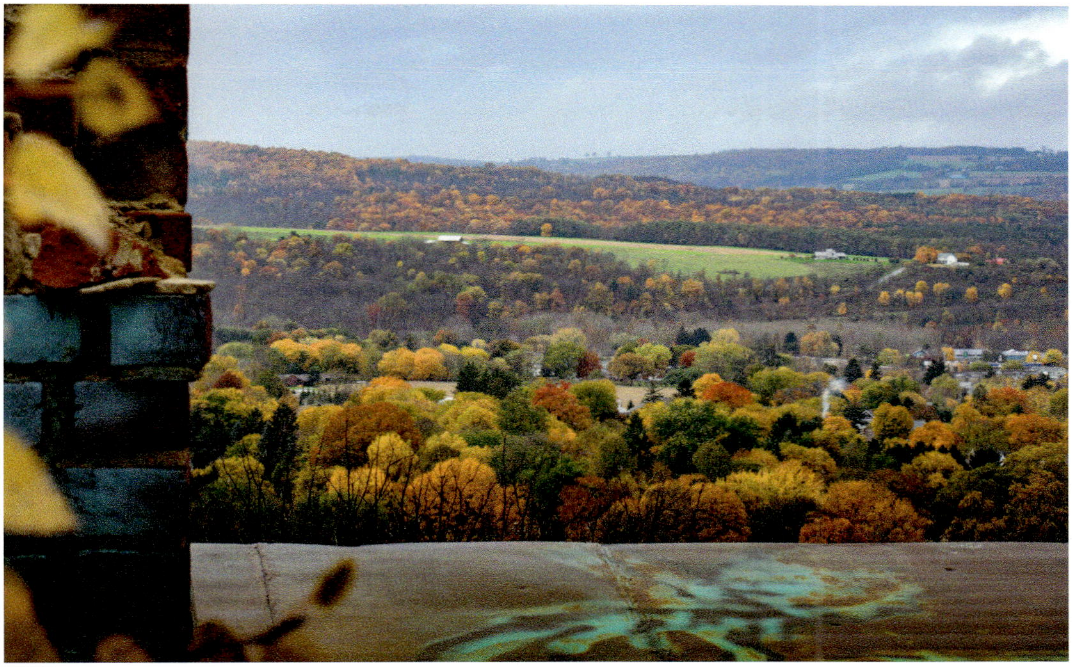

Beyond the crumbling rooftop, the foliage strikes the landscape with autumn colors rolling endlessly for miles. I can only fathom the peaceful pleasure of basking in such beauty as a patient in her heyday. *[Photo by Brian Cray]*

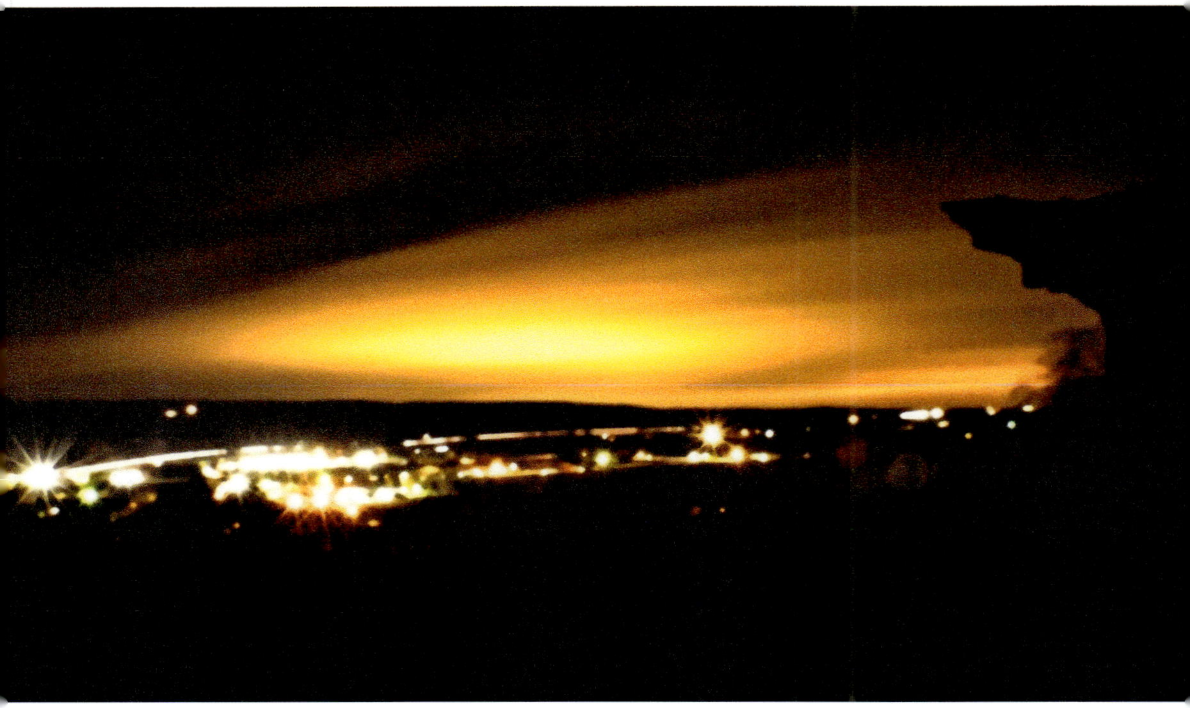

A fiery blaze ignites the sky as I rub my eyes from the rooftop and look out at the big city lights of Dansville. A silhouette of a tower stands in the corner and my eyes droop back to sleep. *[Photo by Brian Cray]*

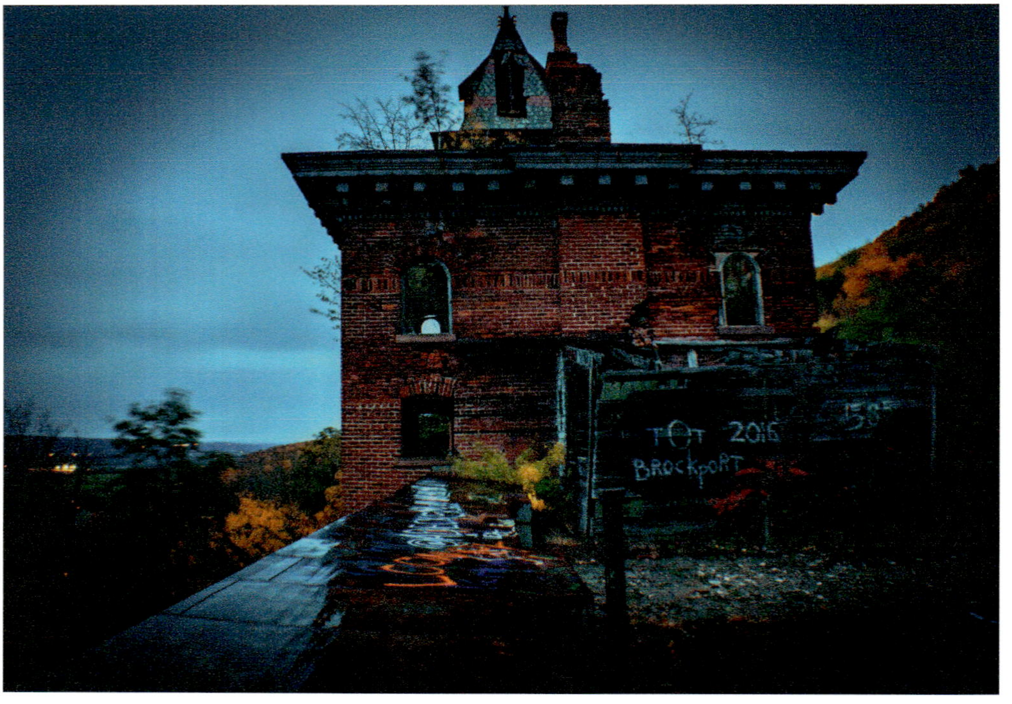

I awake to the pitter of raindrops upon my brow and capture the eerie presence of night fading into day. I follow the sleek metal scribbled with graffiti to Dr. Jackson's office. *[Photo by Brian Cray]*

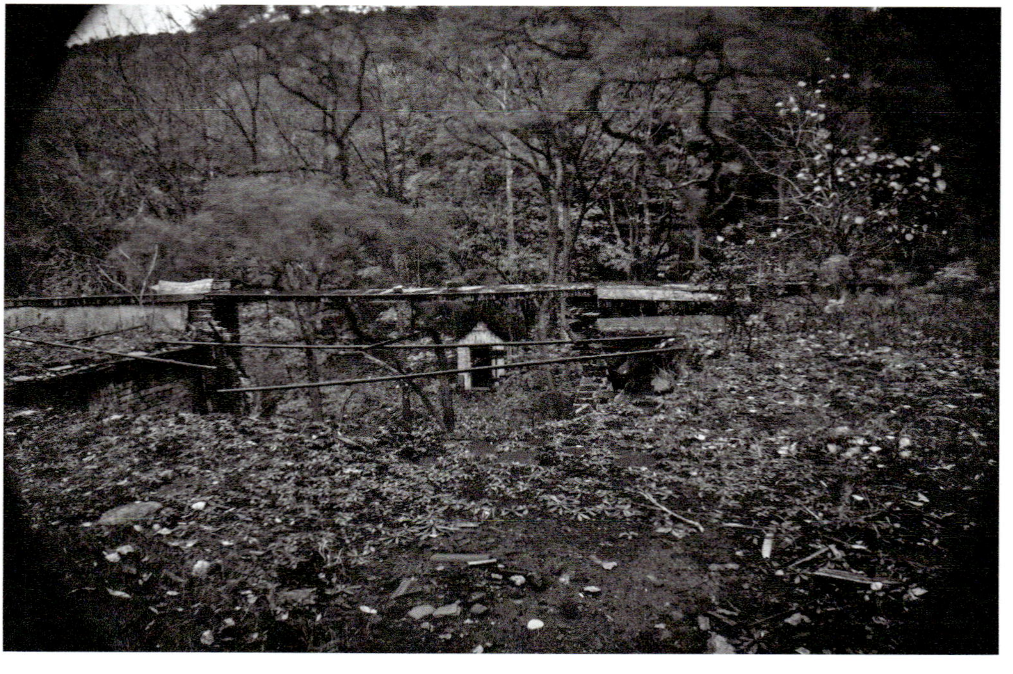

Macfadden founded a religion, Cosmotarianism, based on Christian doctrines and exercise. (Adams, 2010) *[Photo by Brian Cray]*

5

QUACKS, CHARLATANS OR BUSINESS PRODIGIES?

Jackson—a pioneer of the world's first breakfast cereal, owner of the largest hydrotherapy institution in the world, abolitionist, women's suffragist, maker of the American Costume, published author of books and magazines, health nut and boisterous leader—always came out on top as an intelligent businessman. Macfadden—a pioneer of bodybuilding, physical fitness and vegetarianism, owner of a publishing empire, and physical culture restaurants—became the quintessential poster child of success. Each respective reign flourished in the hands of equally qualified yet vastly different men who shared many of the same ideologies and principles on health and fitness, among diet and the sexual organism. They transplanted Sylvester Graham's vegetarian roots to introduce healthier alternatives to pork and beef during the onslaught of the obesity epidemic, which had set its roots between 1870 and 1914, and that advocated natural methods and hydrotherapeutic practices to cure diseases and ailments.[1] Their unorthodox practices have received high criticism over the years despite their entrepreneurial and financial successes. So are Jackson and Macfadden quacks? Are they swindling charlatans or are they just tenacious entrepreneurs running wild with the fresh crazes of the late 1800s and early 1900s?

Jackson asserted that proper diet "cured" masturbation. He maintained such contemptuous feelings throughout his life against medicine so much that he blatantly referred to it as "poison" throughout his published works, particularly in *The Sexual Organism and Its Healthful Management*.[2]

He publicly shunned physicians prescribing medicine to patients and referred to them as "quacks."[3] He touted grandiose claims, one such suggesting that his American Costume rejuvenated women to full health almost immediately upon entering the sanatorium, as seen in a brochure where he touts:

> they have come to us having tried remedies of drug-medicating schools, having gone to other water cures with no benefit, but upon being under our regimen, and adopting the American Costume, they immediately began to get well.
>
> Jackson & Austin, 1871, p. 91

One might yell quackery. The irony behind his statement is that he copied the design of the American Costume off the Bloomer, stating he created the garment two years prior, despite having any substantial proof, merely jumping on a trendy phase for profits through the use of his clever words.[4] This is not the only time he self-promoted his cure-all abilities for financial gain.

Hydrotherapy facilities were a fad of the late 1800s and a product of society's lack of knowledge in the scientific and medical sector for that time period. Jackson, despite possessing an MD, and studying medicine at university, healed patients purely on the placebo effect and through common hygienic practices, which he deemed "psycho-hygienic" in order to substantiate his living. Any success story from his natural methods and hydrotherapeutic work he plastered with media coverage and through constant self-promotion by advertisements in books, brochures, magazines, and newspapers to extend public outreach to the Jackson Sanatorium, but rarely do we stumble upon any of his failures.

> Founded on a rock. For suffering ones and weary
> A home, secure from worldly care and strife,
> Nature, the healing mistress, tends its portals,
> Beckoning with gentle hand to paths of life.
>
> K. J. J.

It is no secret that James Caleb Jackson and his family spent a good portion of their lives in Dansville tending to their business at the Jackson Sanatorium, aiding patients to a righteous path of healthy living, while reaping huge financial success and much prestige as one of the leading hydrotherapy institutions in the world. Despite his criticism and unorthodox eccentricities as a medical practitioner in the late 1800s, without his odd-ball ingenuity, and "chasing the crazes" of the mid- to late century, whether a quack or a swindling charlatan, I do believe his unorthodoxy contributed much to the sanatorium's success through his lectures and beliefs. His vegetarian roots launched the beginning of breakfast cereals spawning from his "Granula" creation. Jackson's beliefs on diet and health also contributed to a following surrounded by raw foodists, and other entrepreneurs adopted his philosophies, extending them to the Midwest, as we see in Battle Creek with Harvey Kellogg and

Ellen White. So despite his self-promoting dribble to reel in paying patrons to his institution, to label him a quack or a charlatan seems unjust. The man held many prosperous qualities as a businessman. His passion and drive contributed to the longevity of the Castle on the Hill, and without his founding of the water cure in 1858, after its many incompetent owners, Dansville would have never frolicked in the memories of such interesting history.

Macfadden boasts equally outlandish claims, proudly wallowing in the "quackery" touted against him, using it as ammunition as he attacks the patented medical field nonstop throughout his lifetime. He preached that drugs were poison, which at that time, with such little research and advancements in medicine, one might reason with him, but critics admonish him for telling his patients not to seek professional physicians. Despite all his outstanding advice as a pioneer of vegetarianism and physical fitness, his quackery also shined when he founded "Cosmotarianism," a religion based on Christianity and physical culture. He also claimed that grape therapy cured cancer and that tugging on one's hair violently each day would prevent them from going bald.[5, 6] The list of his absurdities continues as he truly believed starvation cured any sickness or disease:

> The first thing I would do to a friend who happened to be ill would be to put a sign in front of him that he could see: 'Food is poison – Don't Eat if You Want to Keep Out of the Cemetery.'
>
> Bernarr Macfadden, *Physical Culture*, June 1916

We can also question his sanity when one of Macfadden's daughters died of a heart problem, he spewed, "It's better she's gone, she would have only disgraced me."[7] Clearly, Macfadden fostered many unusual qualities, always looking to capitalize off some aloof business idea to make a buck, which we see through his many rejected health articles, failed business attempts, and mixed array of jobs, along with stints of unemployment. After all, Macfadden adopted his physical culture ideas and publishing empire off of Eugen Sandow's bodybuilding demonstrations. He imitated the same poses and photographed himself with a black cabinet behind his naked flexed body, only covering his appendage with a fig-leaf, which was Sandow's signature pose.[8] Macfadden even copied Sandow's magazine titled *Physical Culture,* releasing it a year after him in America, which advanced Macfadden into a successful career.[9] He also cornered the market in the health spa craze, opening up countless sanatoriums across the nation before finally settling on a gold mine in Dansville, where he made patients believe he could cure them of all sickness through natural means in just eight to twelve weeks. When cereals became the fad of the century, he sprung right up again with Strengthfude, a high-enriched fiber cereal similar to "Granula" and Kellogg's "Granola," but it never took off because of its laxative qualities.[10]

Macfadden chased the next craze and although the Castle on the Hill was not an integral part of his life (he did not live in Dansville) or to his fame and fortune, without his revitalizing the building after the Jackson reign, it would have inevitably sequestered to a debilitating skeleton of forgotten memories much earlier on in its history. His passion, eccentricities and principles sprang life to an otherwise defunct water cure, revamping it to the talk of the town at the Sugar Bowl amongst the locals. The health resort employed a generation of workers. It brought celebrities, patrons and curious souls, sneaking around the premises to peek at the naked sunbathers on the roof. Airplanes even circled at low altitudes to creep in on the action. Teenagers snuck into the pool at night and got into mischief. It became a symbol of the town and his presence may have been forgotten elsewhere around the world, but not in Dansville. He employed happiness, and a cult following of health enthusiasts who live by his very words even to this day. Just browse Reddit if you don't believe me. For that, he is not only a mastermind behind the propulsion of physical fitness, but also one of two hard-working, unorthodox men, who gave the small town of Dansville a taste of a national presence.

Is he a quack, a charlatan or a senile old man? Body Love is probably a little of each, but regardless of his outlandish claims, his homoerotic and risqué magazines, and his narcissistic obsession with his own body, his presence lives on as the founding father of physical culture and the small town of Dansville will never forget him or his contributions. Much like Jackson, he died a legend, with enough clout to warrant criticism from those who opposed his beliefs. I am sure he is smiling, doing push-ups and dumbbell curls in his grave, peddling "Weakness is a crime" from the heavens.

Today, the brick Victorian castle slumps on the hill, overlooking Dansville, and with each passing harsh winter, its crumbling base, distressed walls, and mangled supports slowly strips away at its history while nearing collapse. A report in January of 2008 by the New York State Restore Communities Initiative allotted $2.5 million for building restoration, but as of my last two visits in 2016 and again in 2018, the castle barely stands with irreparable structural damage, making the site both an eyesore and inherent danger to the community.[11] Layers of thick dust and dirt pile in its corners. Bits of brick lay in heaps of rubble at its teetering base, opening the scars of its empty walls to water damage and continued beatings by Mother Nature.

In 2001, Peter Krog, owner of the Buffalo-based real estate development firm Krog Corp., took ownership of the property, but after eighteen years, the Castle on the Hill continues to rot away, year after year, with its only deterrent a “No Trespassing” sign plastered to its kicked-in, plywood doors.[12] Dansville Police Department estimate about forty trespassing charges a year are handed out, and it is only a matter of time until this structure completely collapses, sending rubble and brick hurling down the hill along Route 256.[13]

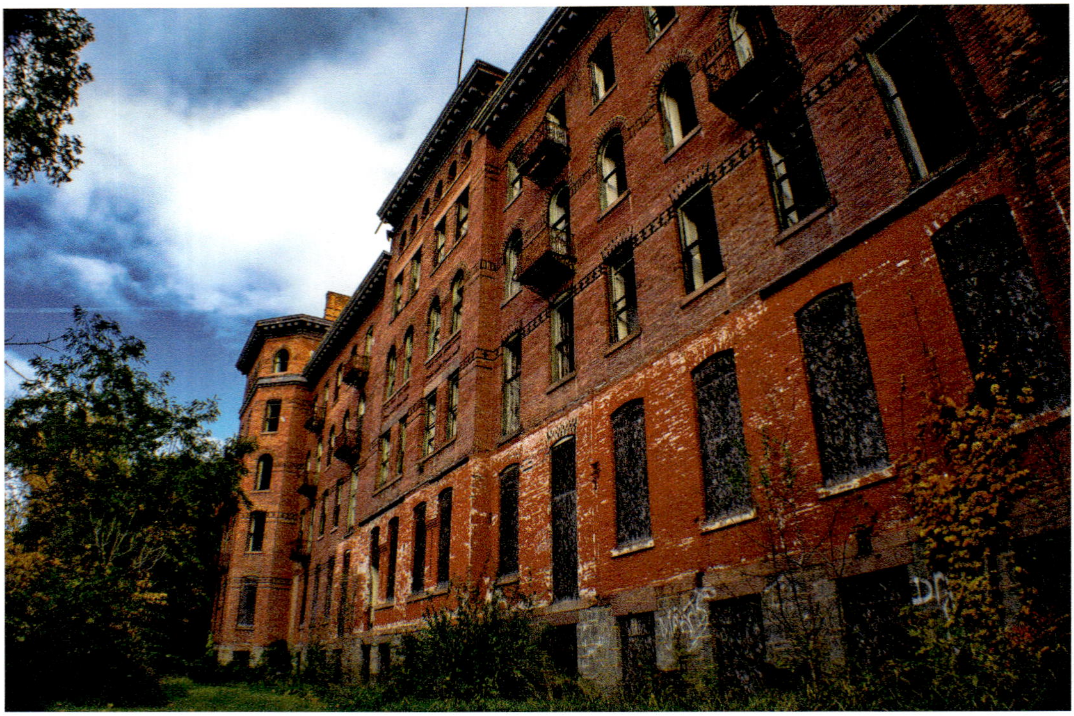

I entered the neglected structure through the front to explore the history left behind. The word "resort" distinguishes a strong distinction between "sanitarium," which limits treatments to incurable diseases, along with mental and tubercular patients. *[Photo by Brian Cray]*

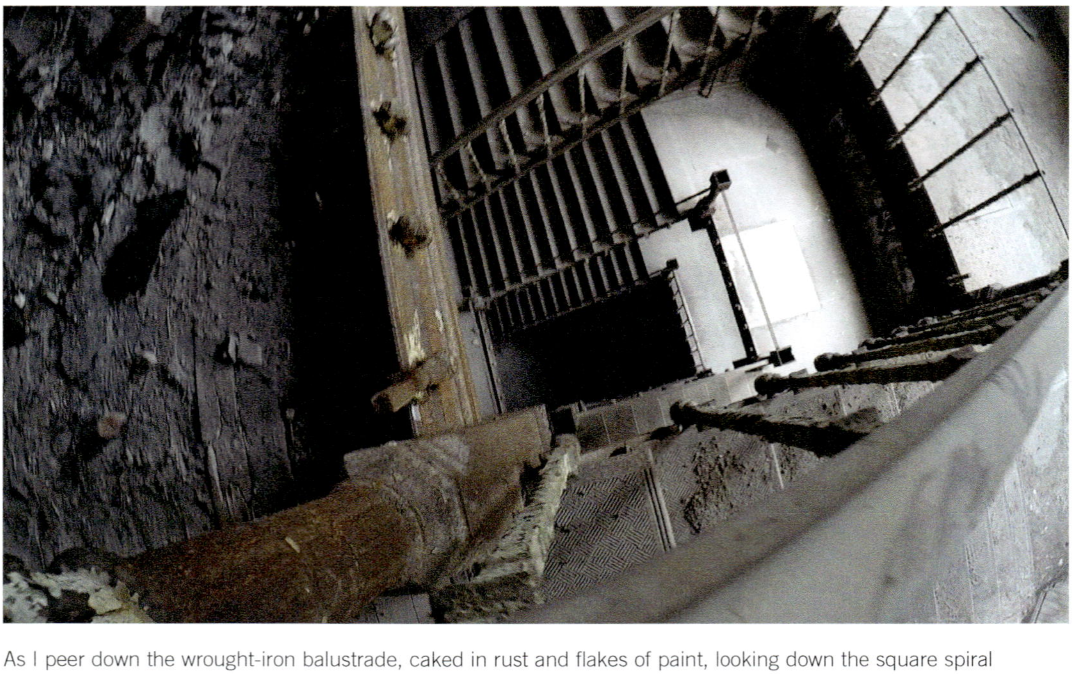

As I peer down the wrought-iron balustrade, caked in rust and flakes of paint, looking down the square spiral staircase, my feet tremble as I get progressively closer to the roof. *[Photo by Brian Cray]*

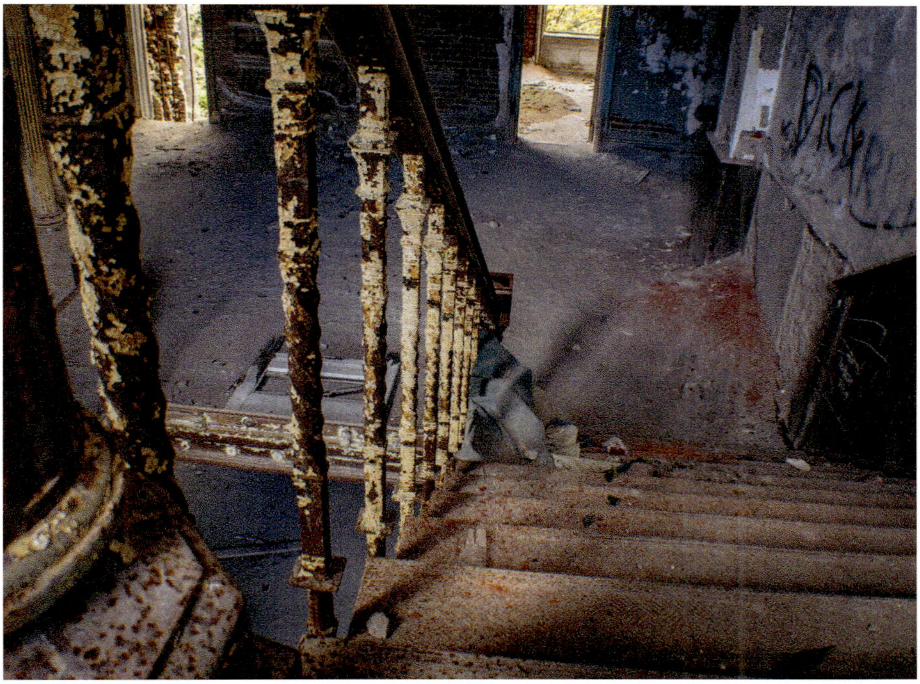

As I peak down the balustrade, freckles of rust brown the railing and steps in momentous decay. *[Photo by Brian Cray]*

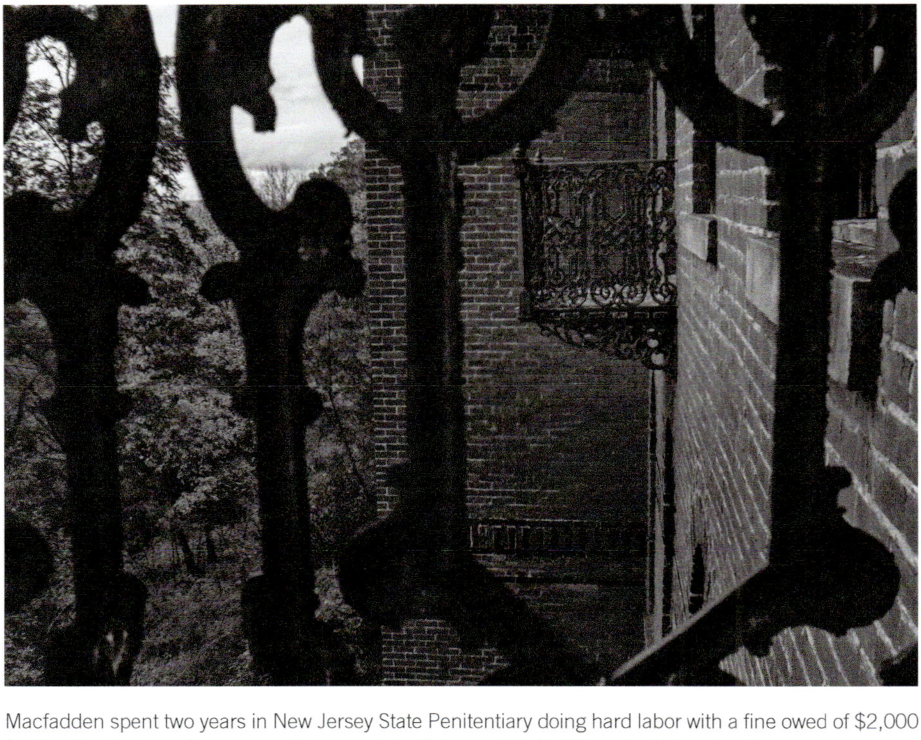

Macfadden spent two years in New Jersey State Penitentiary doing hard labor with a fine owed of $2,000 for the distribution of pornographic materials. (Adams, 2010) *[Photo by Brian Cray]*

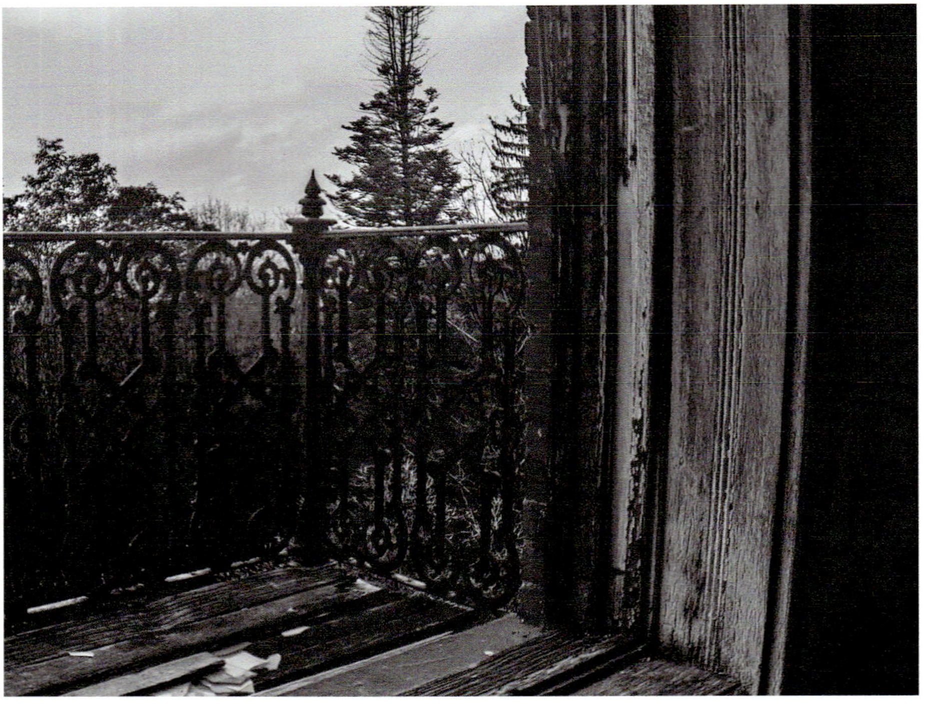

Macfadden called white bread “the staff of death.” (Adams, 2010) *[Photo by Brian Cray]*

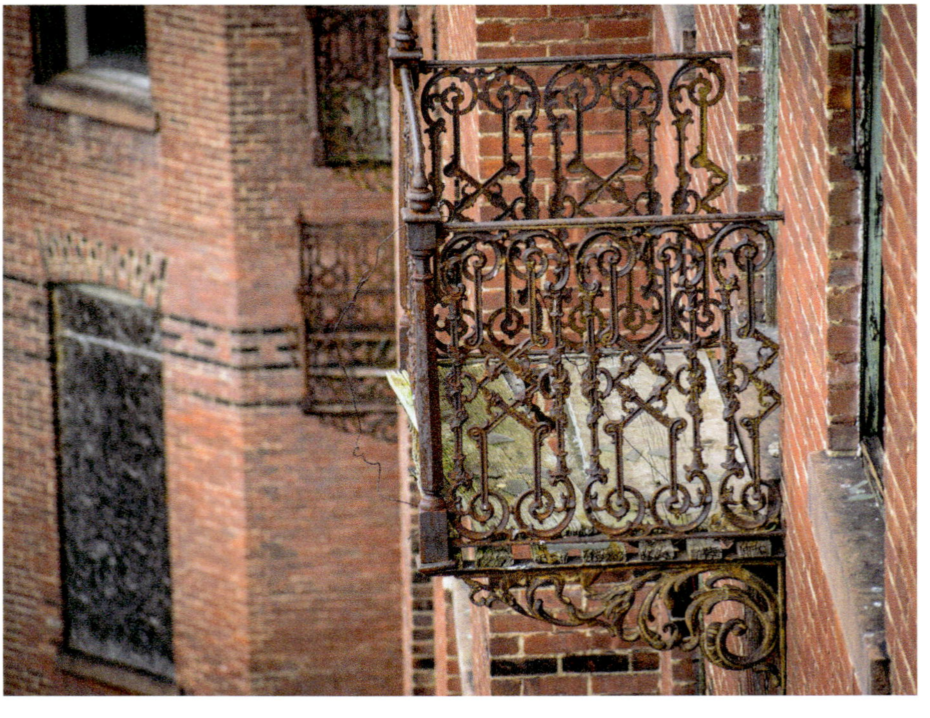

Her iron twists and curves like withered vines, browning through the depths of time, holding onto her crimson walls with her last bits of strength. *[Photo by Brian Cray]*

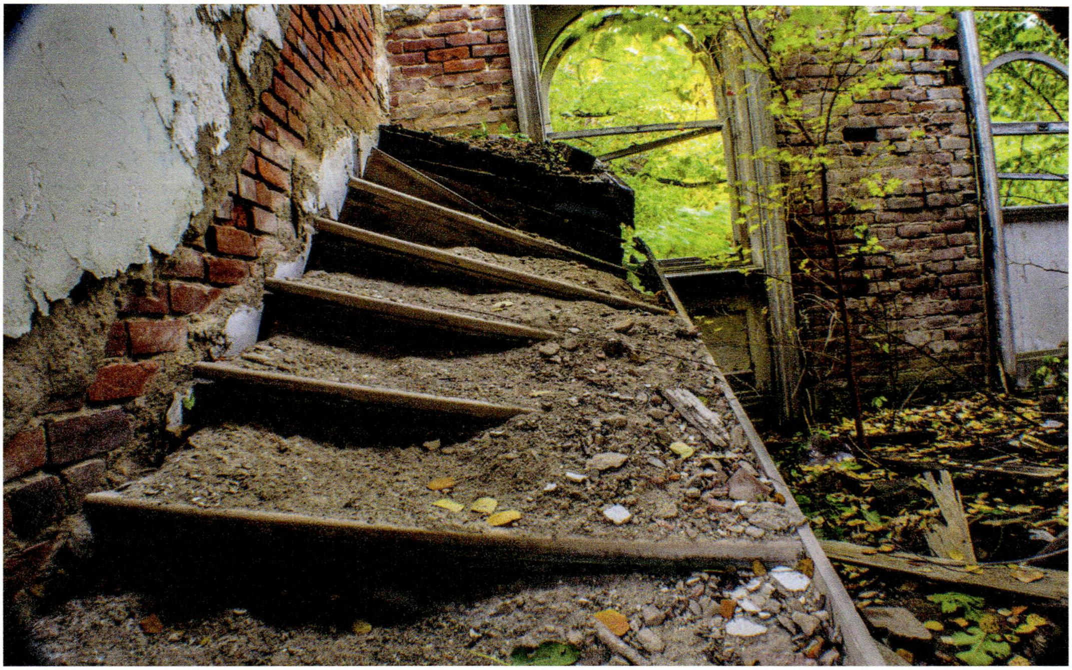

Stairs lead to nowhere with years of dust piling in the corners of each step. At one point in time, they led to the roof of the tower for sunbathers. *[Photo by Brian Cray]*

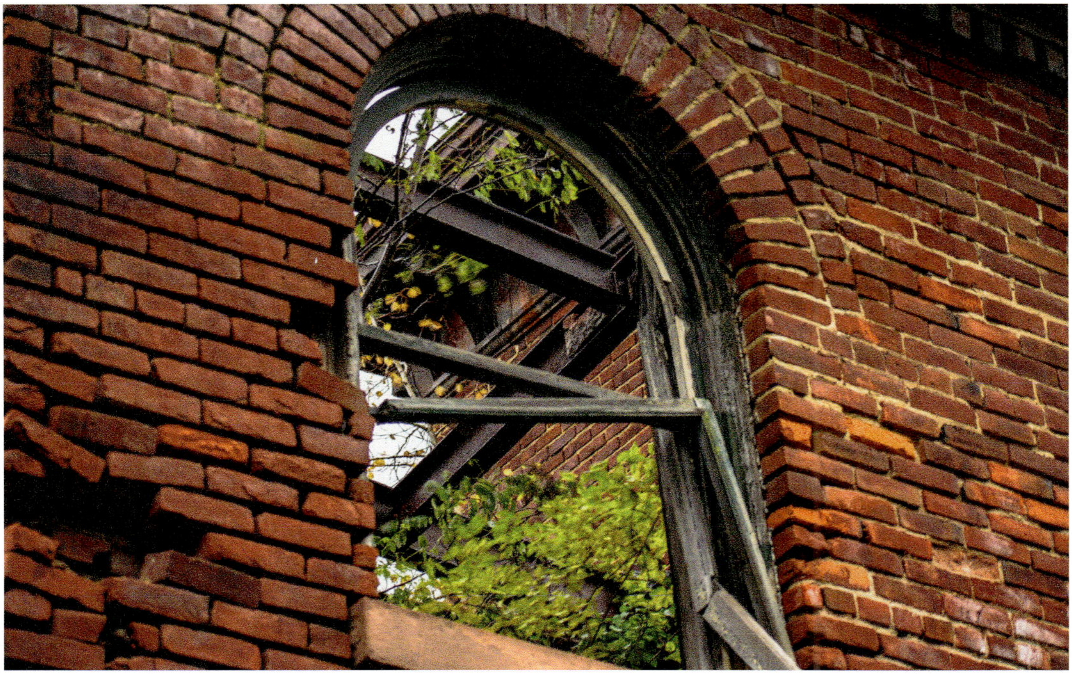

The new building had a basement and five stories. The basement held the laundry, bakery, sewing room, and dining room for helpers, storage facilities and a vault, all of which are no longer accessible because of its current state of decay. (Jackson, 2010) *[Photo by Brian Cray]*

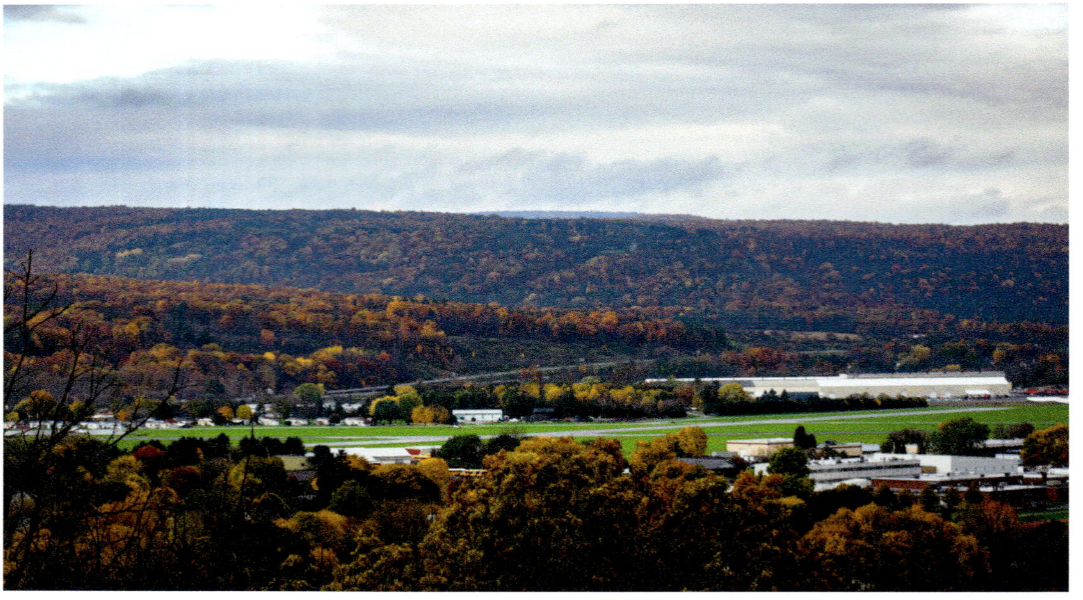

In the distance, I can see the airfield for Dansville airport where pilots would take off and fly by the castle to peek at the sunbathers on the rooftop of the P.C. *[Photo by Brian Cray]*

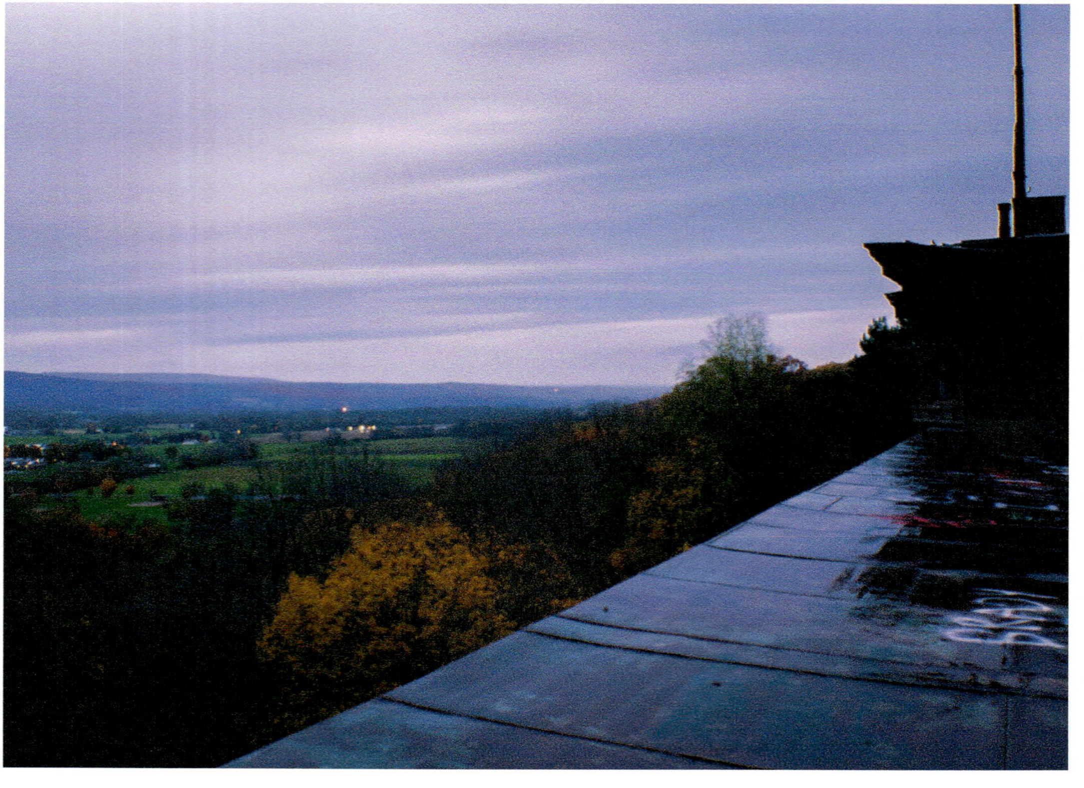

As the sun pokes out behind the clouds, the rain stops briefly and I wander towards the dance floor to explore more of the roof. *[Photo by Brian Cray]*

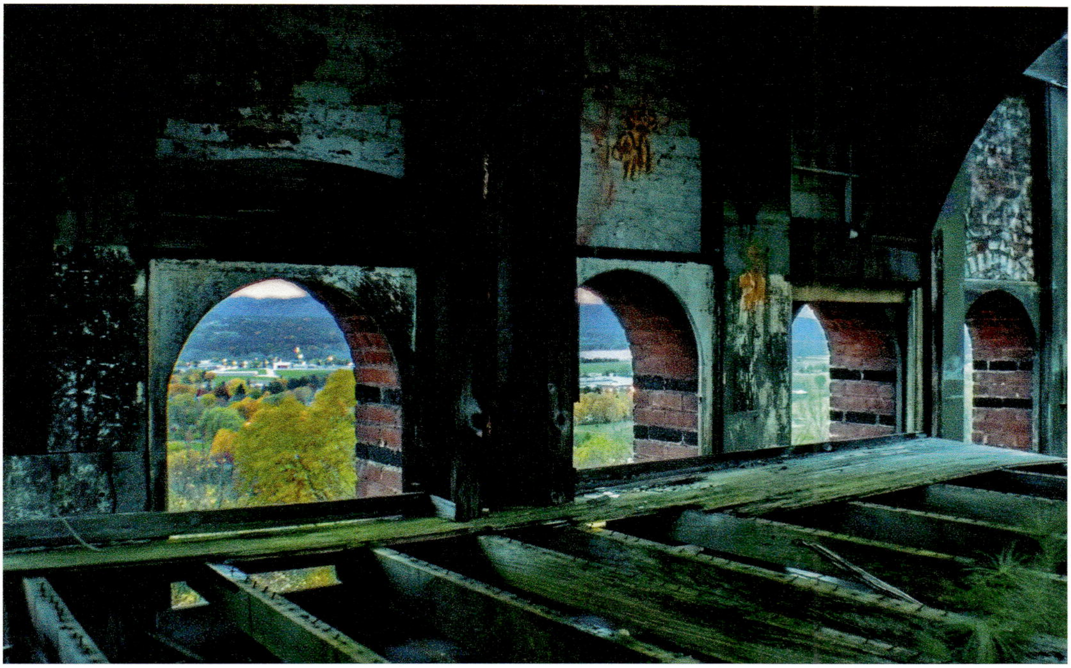

Painted windows of fall dwindle as my eyes wander the narrowing arches behind the dance floor. *[Photo by Brian Cray]*

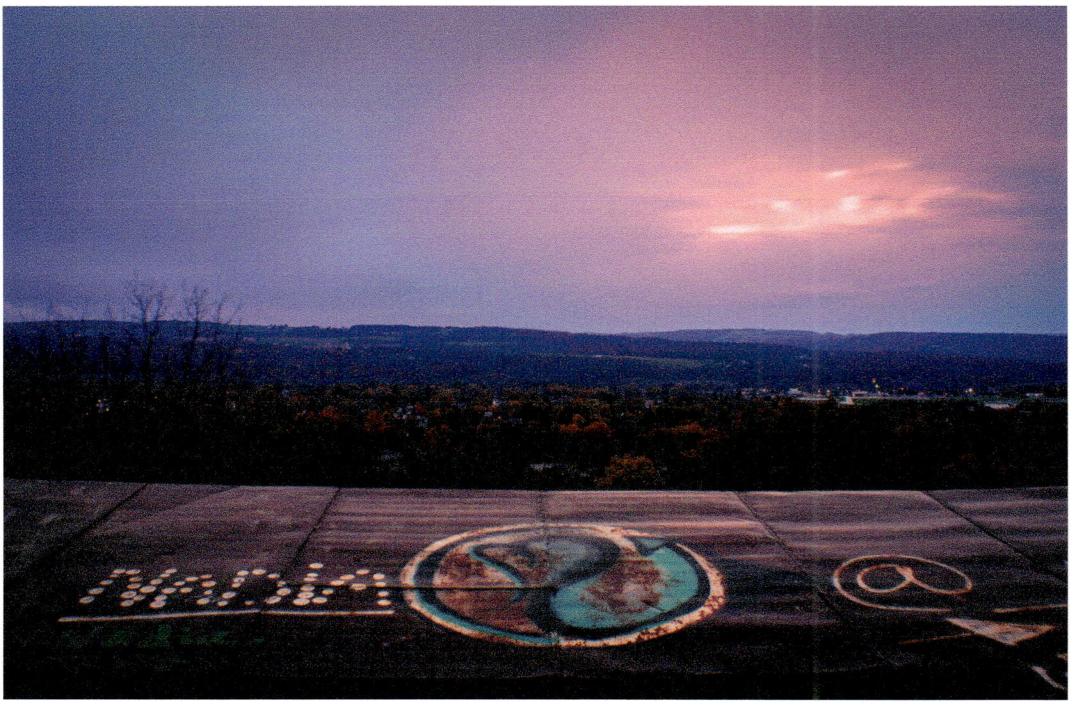

Pink lemonade melts the sky as my eyes stick to the words "NADIA" wandering off to the circular disk drizzled in black, white and blue. *[Photo by Brian Cray]*

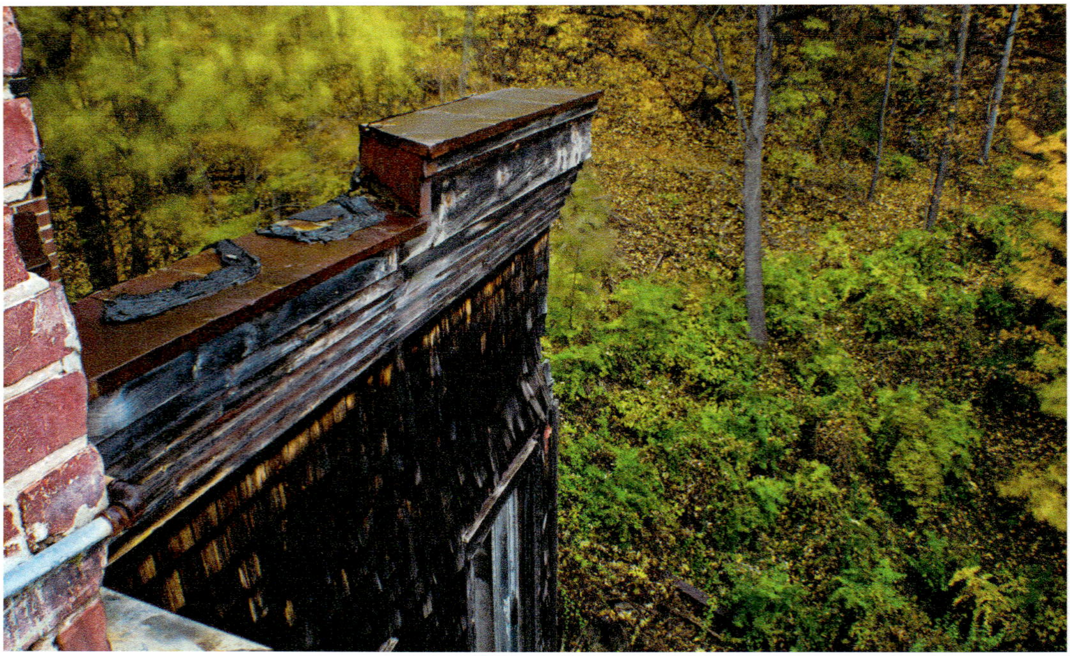

Wispy tree branches blur vibrantly behind charred flaps of wooden shingles flapping in the wind. *[Photo by Brian Cray]*

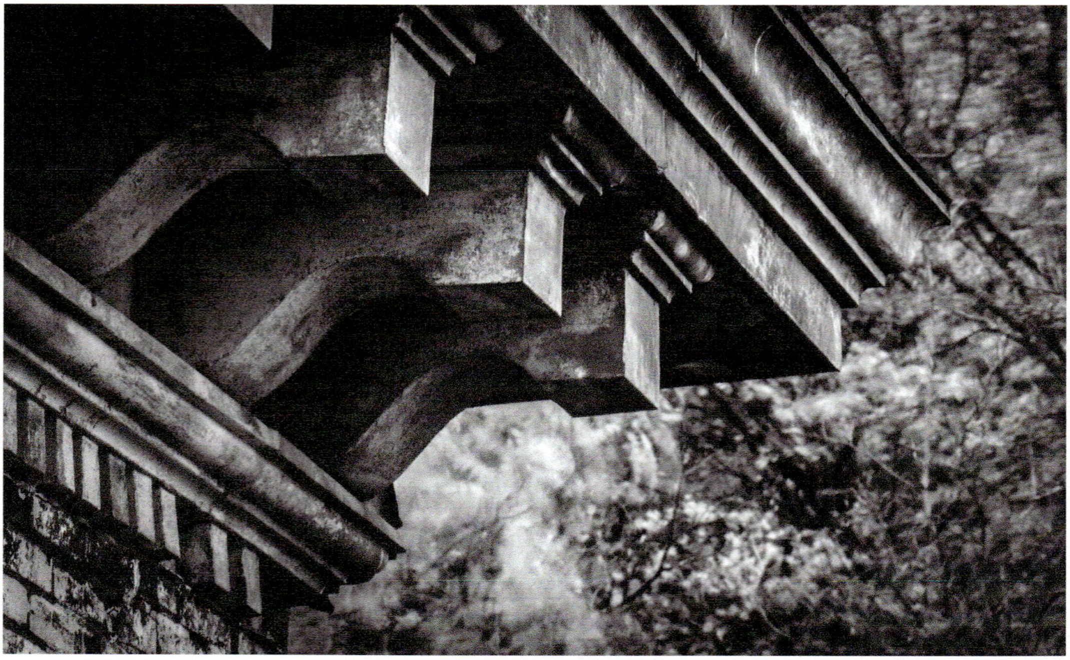

Did you know Macfadden met with Mussolini in Italy and when he went to clasp his hand in a firm shake, "Your soldiers eat too much" catapulted from Macfadden's mouth uncontrollably? He offered to show off his physical culture knowledge and Mussolini accepted, sending forty cadets to the sanatorium the following year. (Adams, 2010) *[Photo by Brian Cray]*

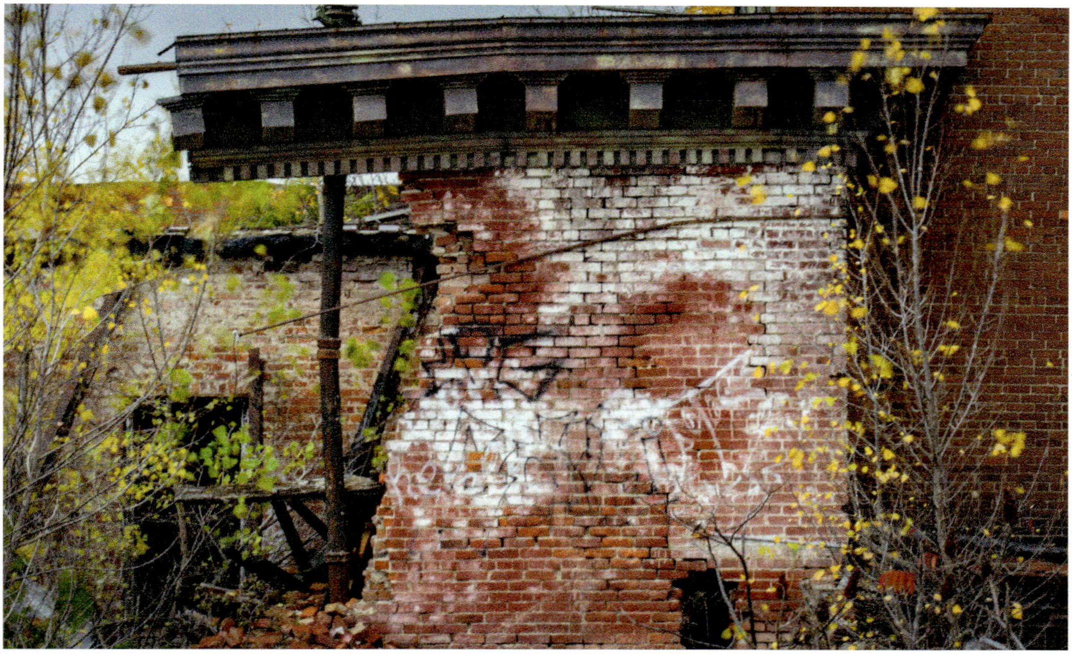

As my eyes zigzag between the narrow voids of brick, I can see where more pieces will shear and join the broken bits of rubble and bent pipes below. *[Photo by Brian Cray]*

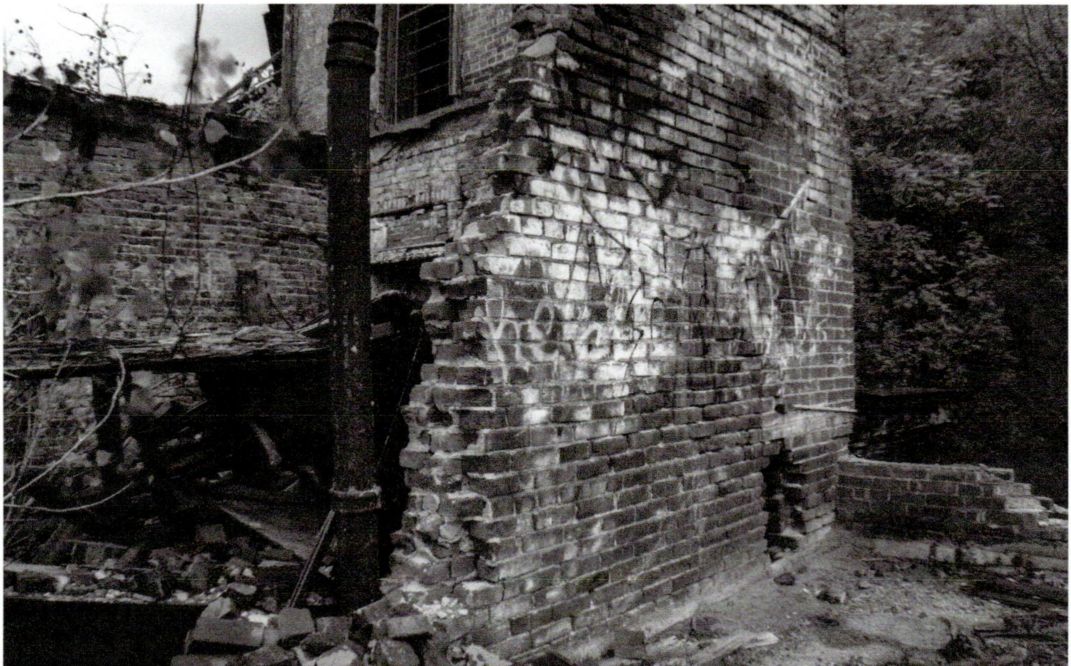

Macfadden and his first wife performed "The Perfect Woman" contest around Europe for the promotion of Physical Culture. His pregnant wife would jump from a table landing onto his stomach. The crowd would "ooohhh" and "aaahhh" and Macfadden would pop up unscathed and bow exuberantly. (Adams, 2010) *[Photo by Brian Cray]*

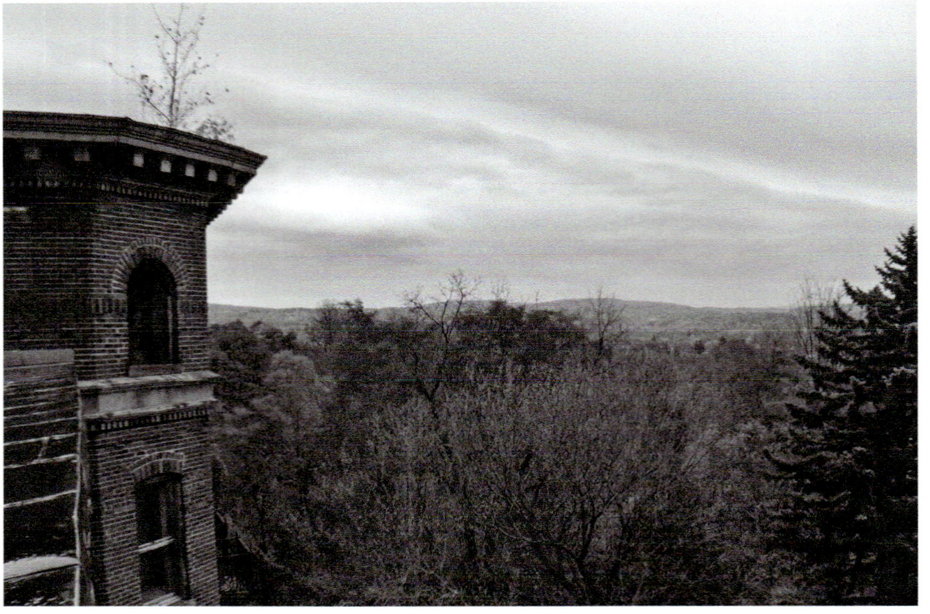

Did you know Macfadden ran for Senate in Florida, and even if he had won the election, he would have been disqualified for not having five years of residency? (Adams, 2010) *[Photo by Brian Cray]*

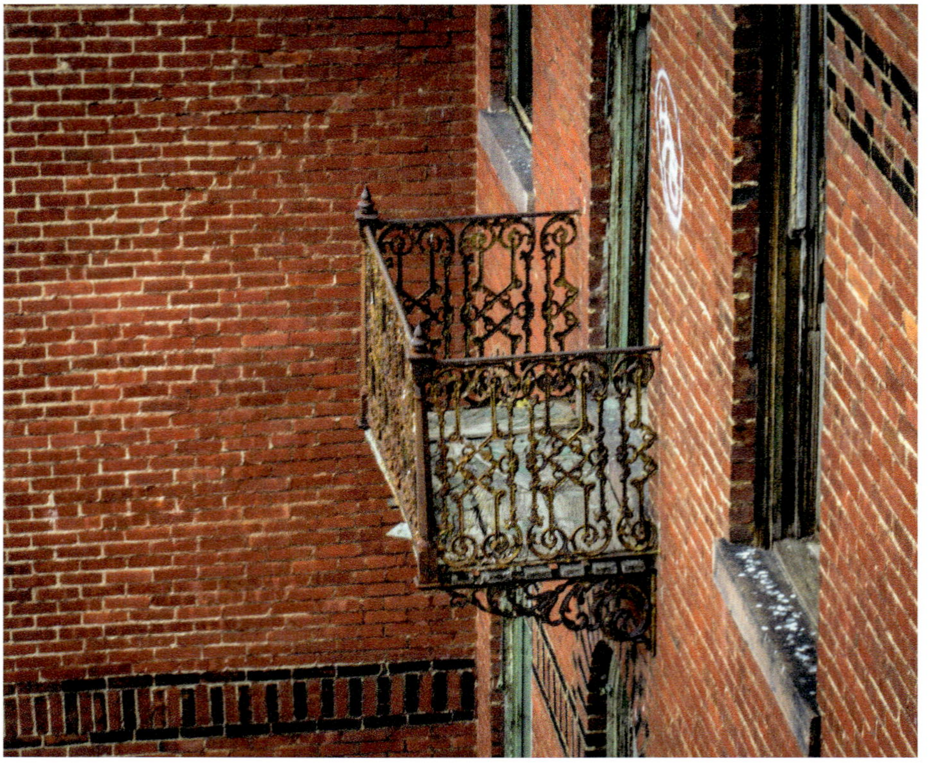

She bleeds a deep red as a victim of time and every balcony clings on to a lost cause. *[Photo by Brian Cray]*

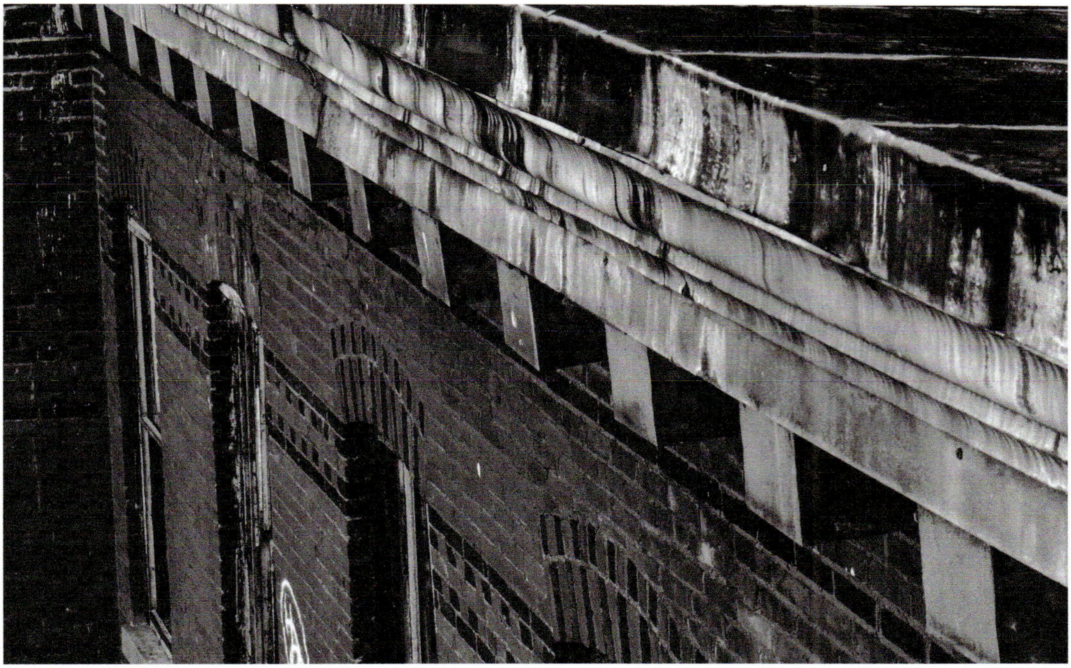

The San attracted patients from a much broader area when the Delaware, Lackawanna and Western Railroad completed its depot in Dansville. Before this, patients rode the train into Wayland and took a stagecoach to Dansville, which was more of an inconvenience. (Jackson, 2010) *[Photo by Brian Cray]*

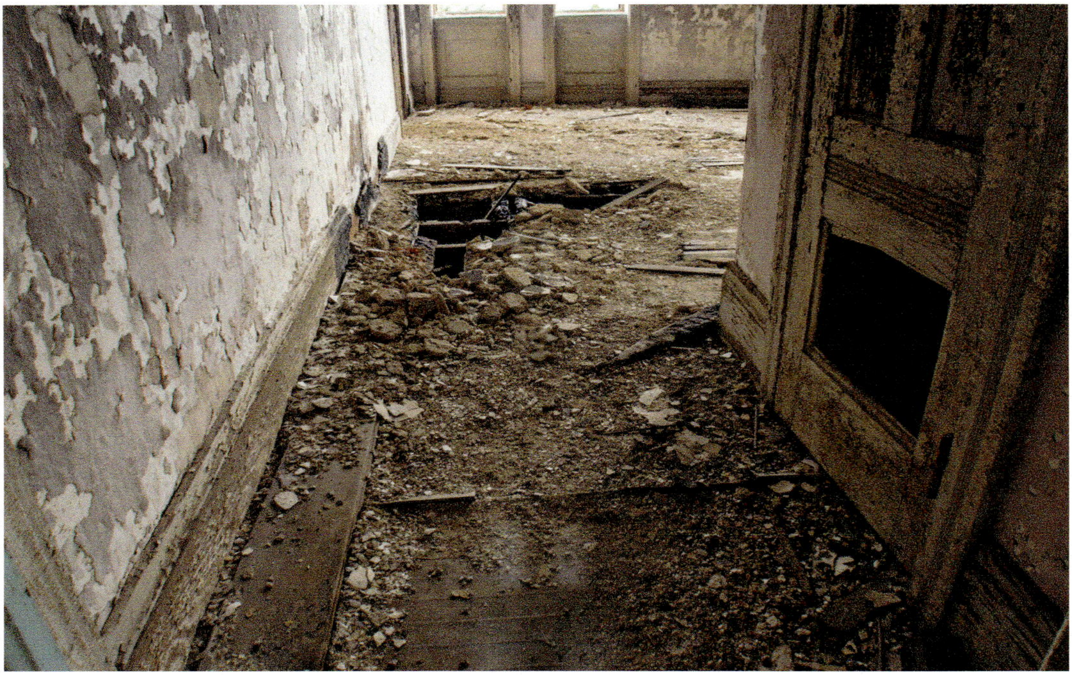

All you will see is crumbled bits of her past as stories fade away within her dying walls. Much of her furniture was sold off after Fromcheck died in 1972 and what remains was left to perish. (Jackson, 2010) *[Photo by Brian Cray]*

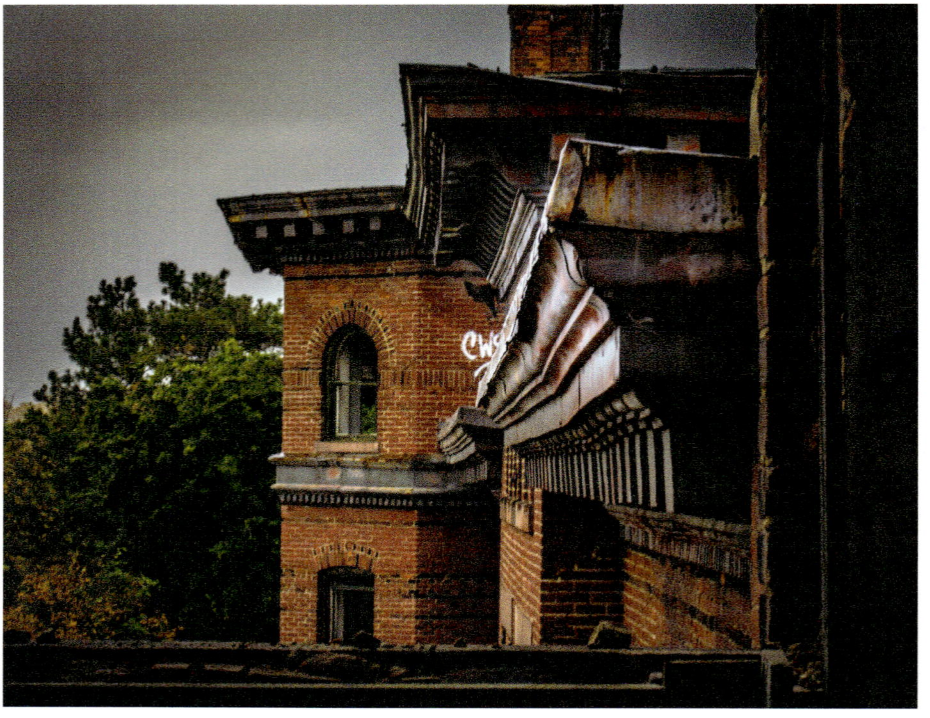

My eyes follow the rusted leading edge of sheet metal across the rooftop to the far club room and I wonder just how many occupants they held in there at a given time. *[Photo by Brian Cray]*

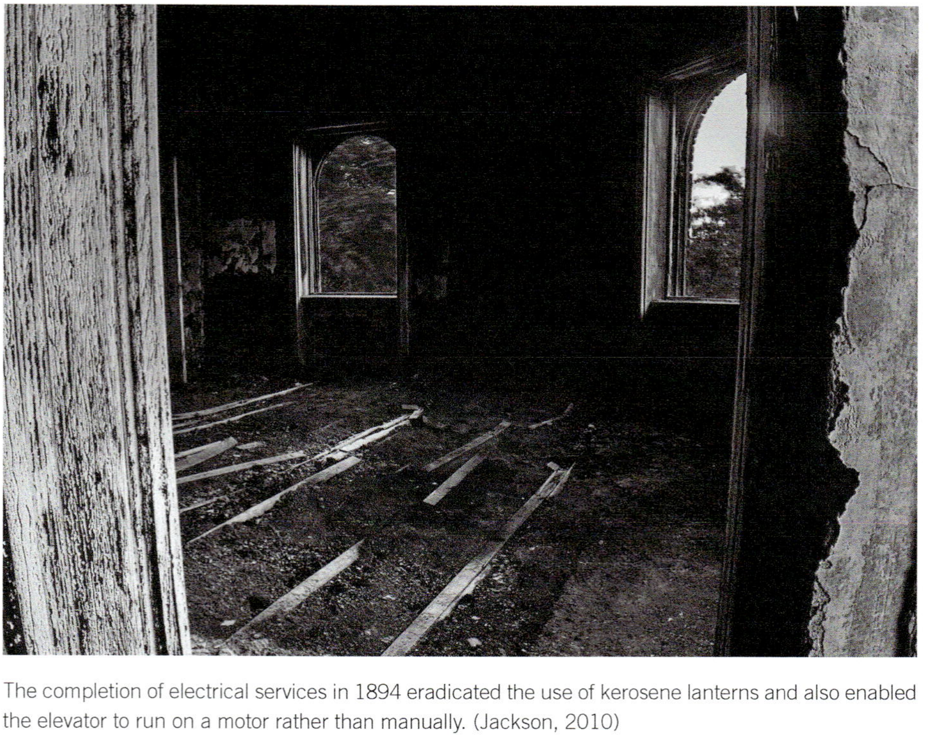

The completion of electrical services in 1894 eradicated the use of kerosene lanterns and also enabled the elevator to run on a motor rather than manually. (Jackson, 2010)

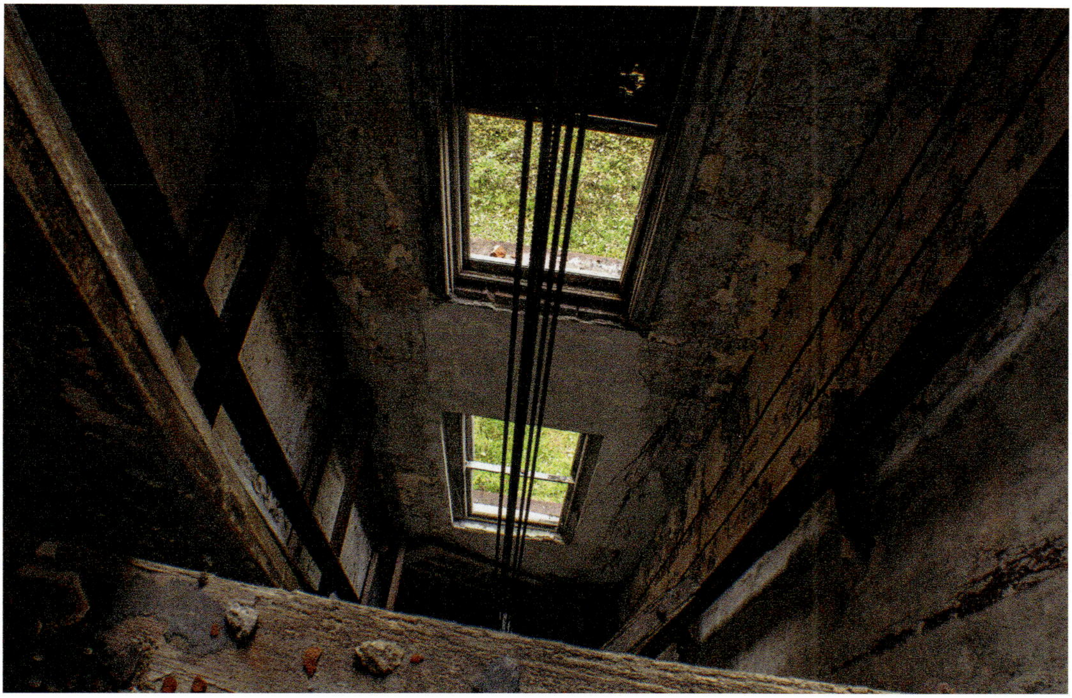

My jittery feet stagger along the slippery rooftop, pittering closer to the open elevator shaft. My heart sinks, spiraling down the tarnished cable, as my eyes tumble to the ground floor to a pit of fractured wood and splintered doors, suffering at the whim of nature.

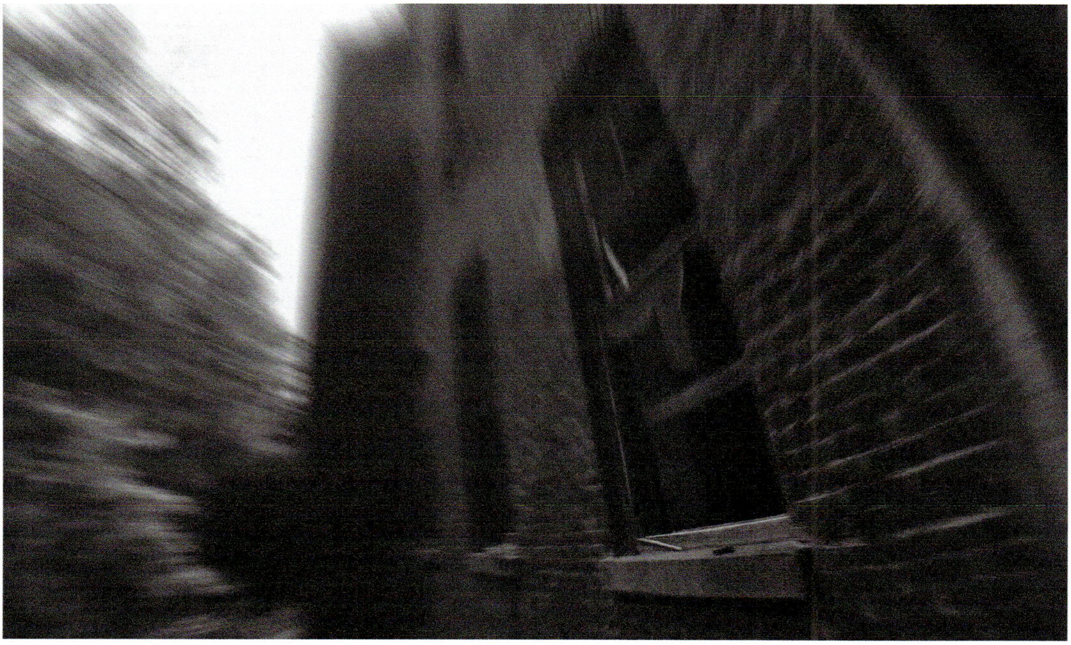

I lean out the splintered windowsill looking out through broken windows at the once vibrant rooms of the Jackson Sanatorium that now lay dark and dismal in their defunct demise.

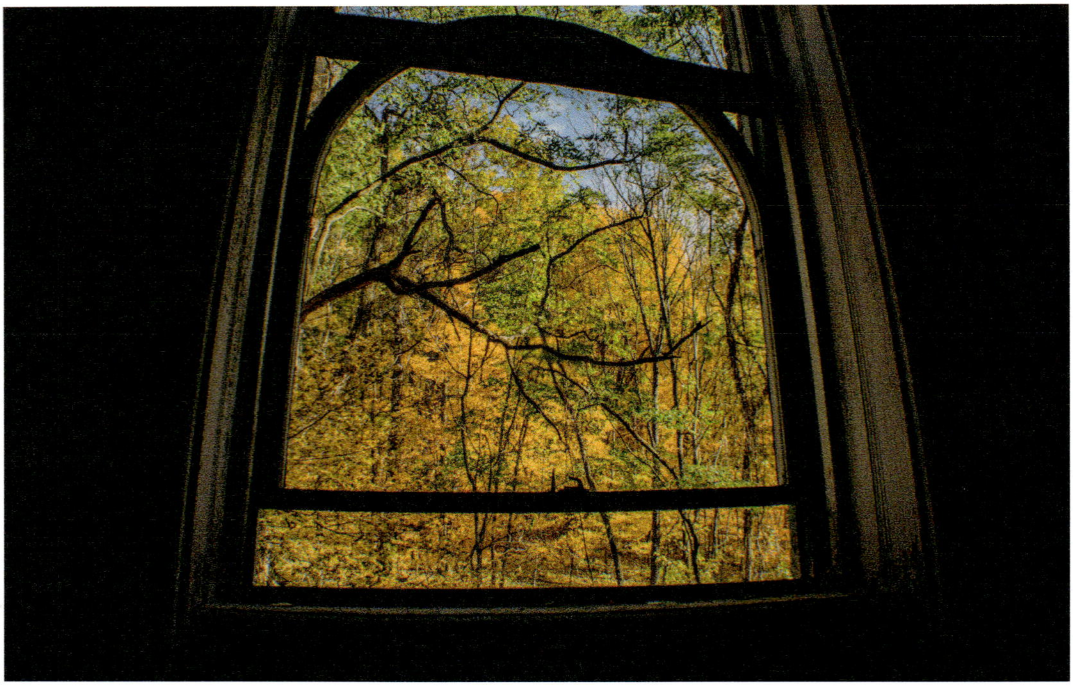

As I stare through the arched window, it feels like I am looking at the vibrant strokes of a paintbrush through the silhouette of canvas.

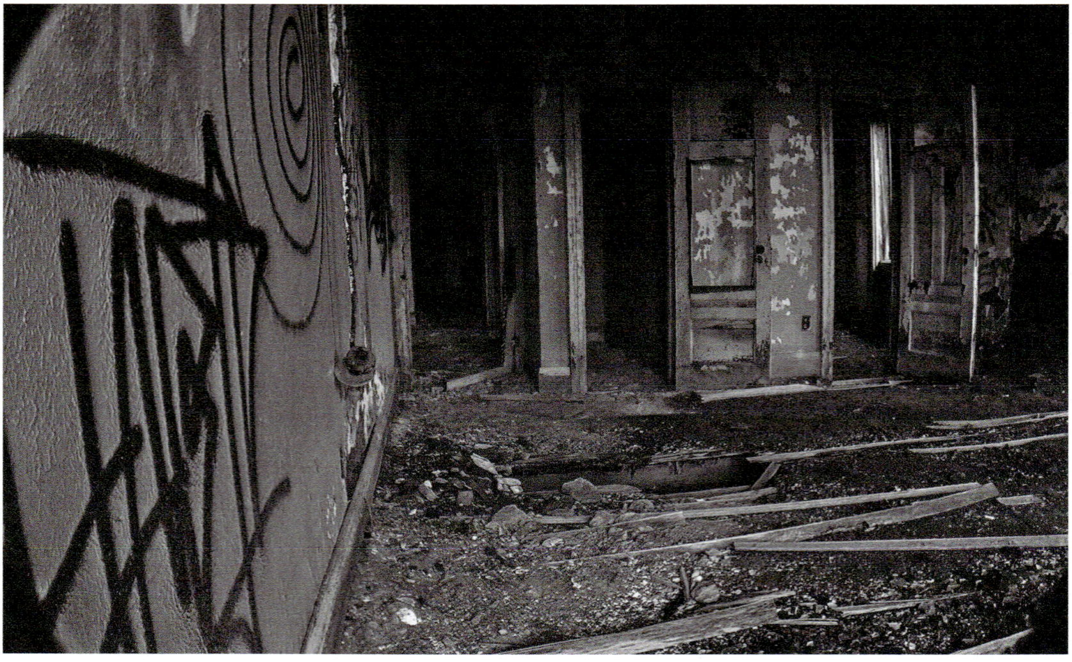

The San had a huge number of "cottages" occupying the east hill, which were small mansions. *Clover Nook, The Terrace, Ivy Lodge, Hollyhock, Alma, Crown Hill,* and *Villula* acted as additional rooms for patients in 1880 with at least ten or more cottages appearing over the next twenty years. (Jackson, 2010)

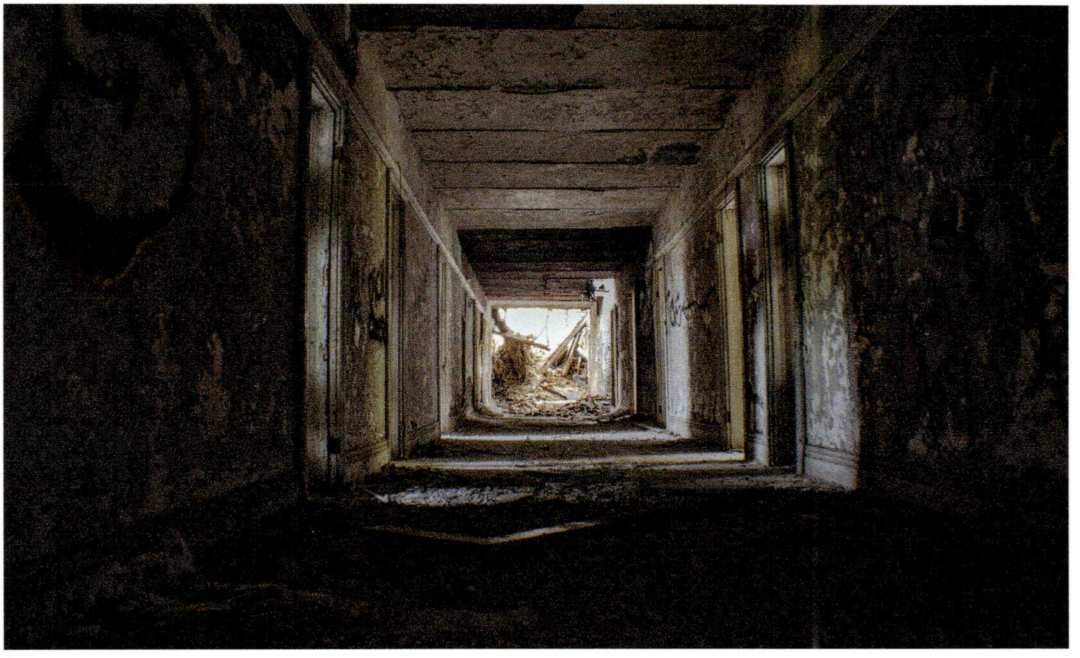

As I look down the corridor, I can see the distress of her walls after thirty-eight years of closure. Paint peels back to her crumbling base with loose doors stacked astray in the hallway. It is only a matter of time before the claws of Mother Nature sink into her scars, ripping her wounds open to a pile of rubble.

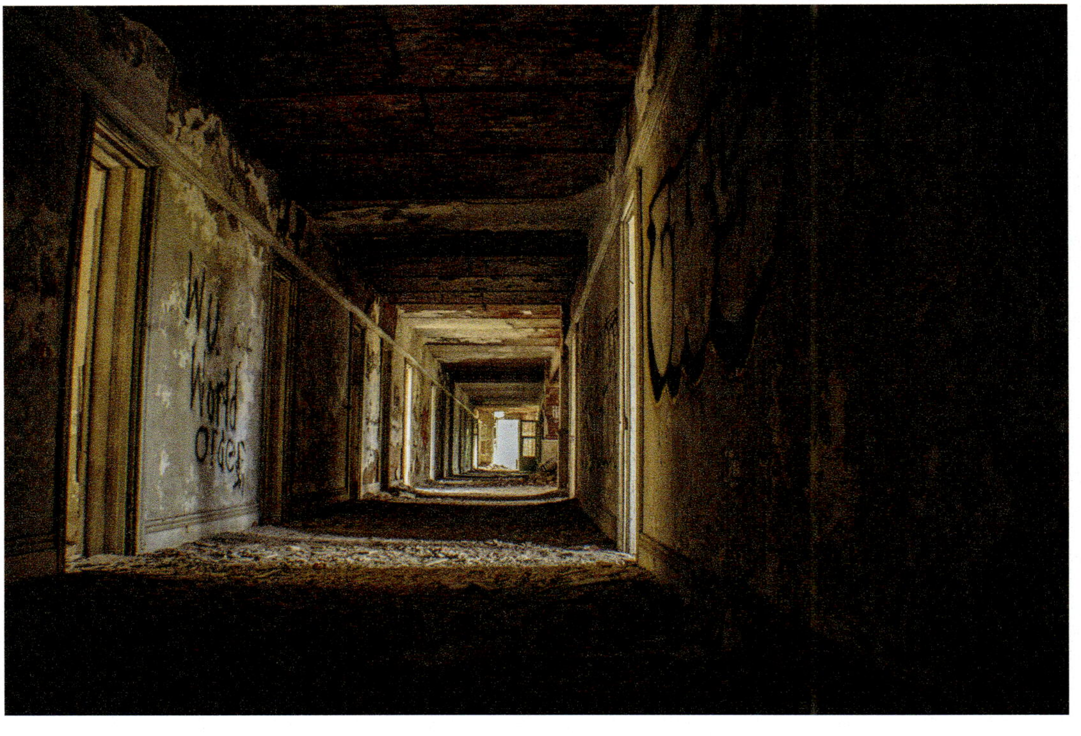

Every hallway tapers off to an end, and as I look into the light, one day I will be there too.

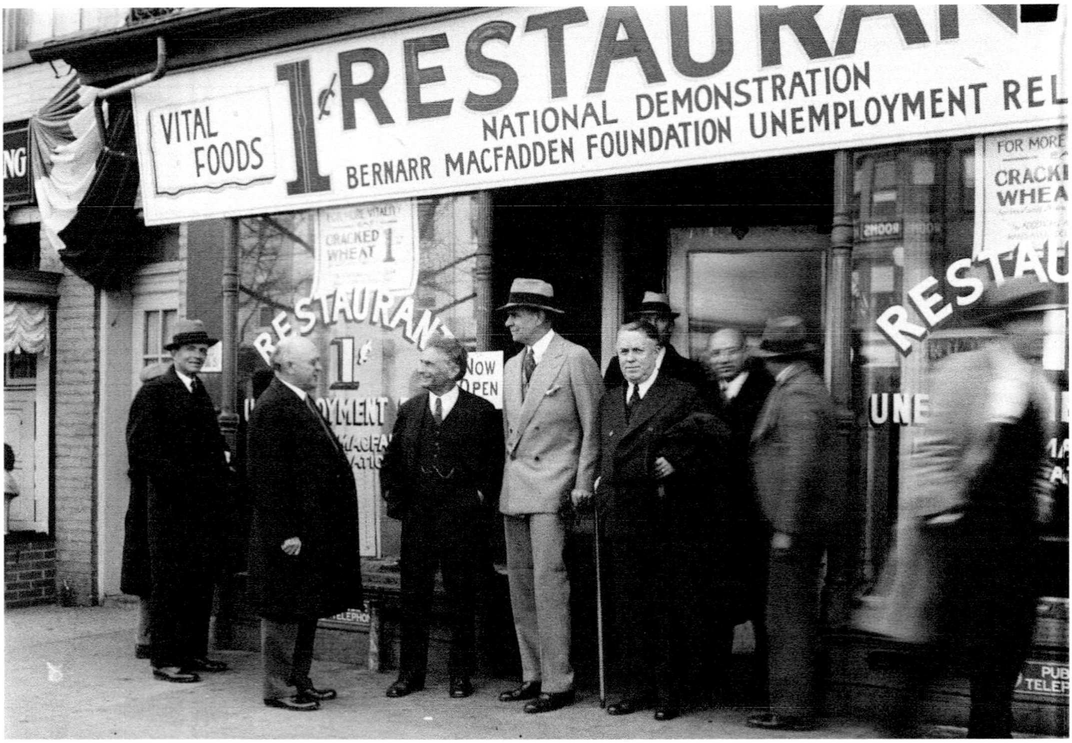

Bernarr Macfadden stands outside of one of his many one-cent restaurants to demonstrate philanthropy for unemployment relief from the Depression. *[Photo by Harris & Ewing, photographer]*

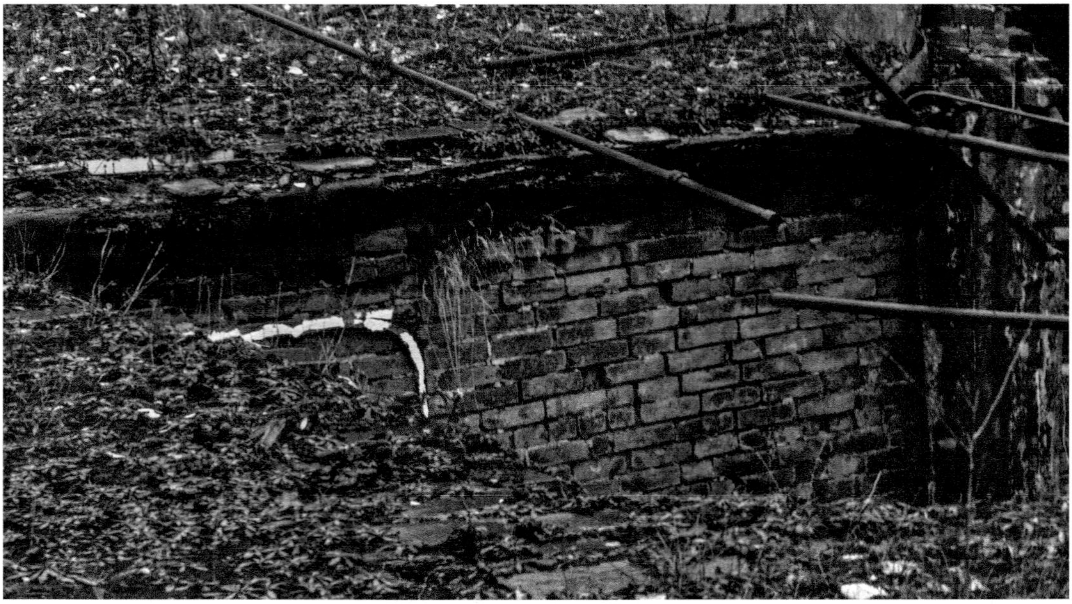

A sinkhole of fallen bricks sits in a graveyard five stories below as I gently creep closer to this deplorable sight, one I have never seen before in my lifetime. The real wrench of The Jackson Health Resort's demise came years ago when the Army moved in after the San declared voluntary bankruptcy. (Jackson, 2010) *[Photo by Brian Cray]*

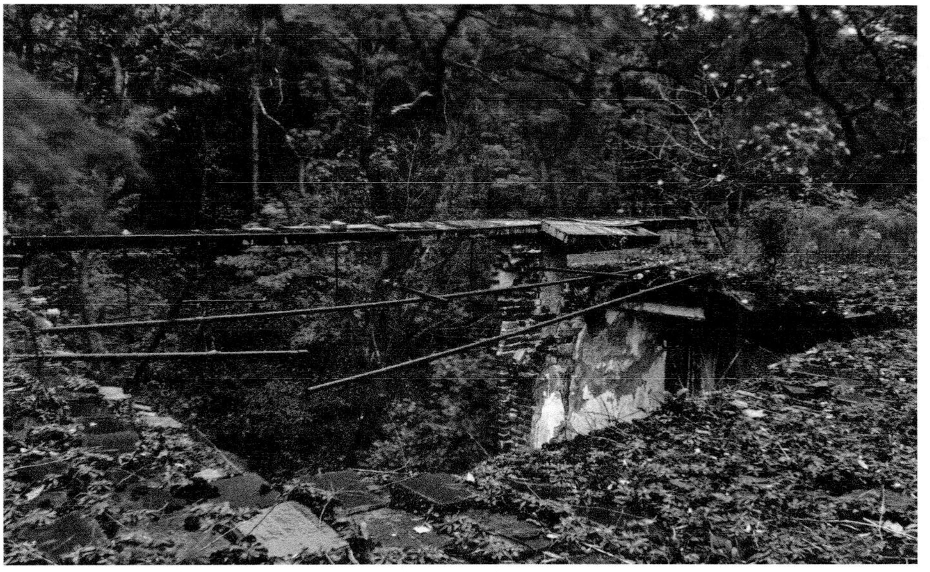

When the Army moved in on February 1, 1918, they only stayed a few months before cancelling their contract and moving to Virginia. Incompetent government personnel damaged the boilers, which no longer produced electricity, but only heat, proving detrimental for the San to regain future operations. (Jackson, 2010) *[Photo by Brian Cray]*

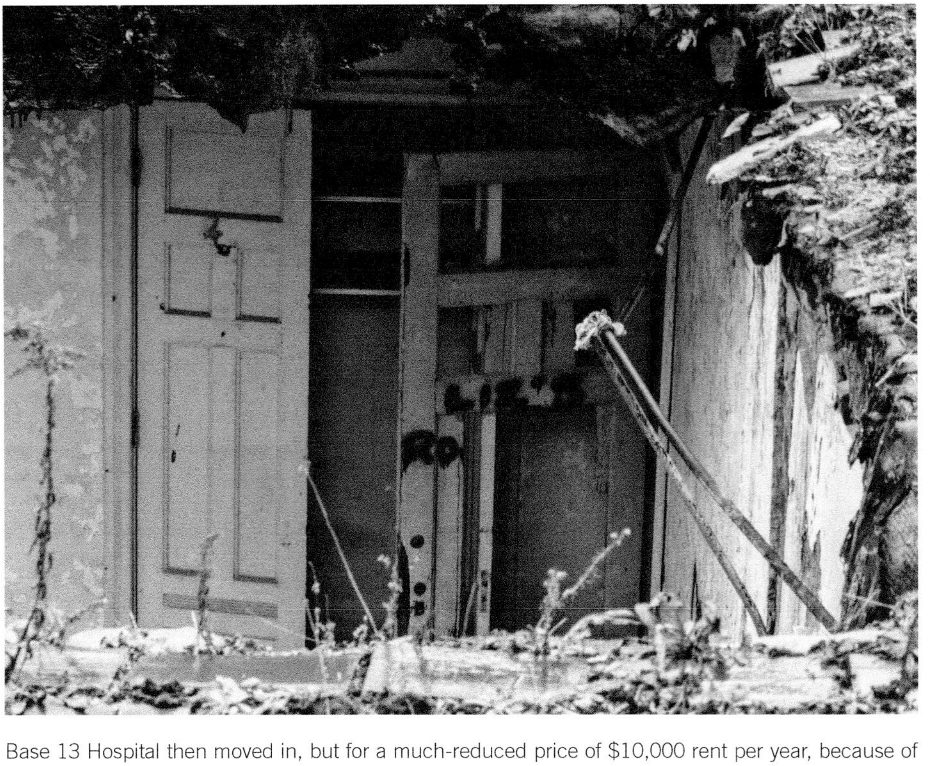

Base 13 Hospital then moved in, but for a much-reduced price of $10,000 rent per year, because of the damages incurred from previous Army personnel. Patients arrived not even two weeks after World War I ended for psychiatric treatment. (Jackson, 2010) *[Photo by Brian Cray]*

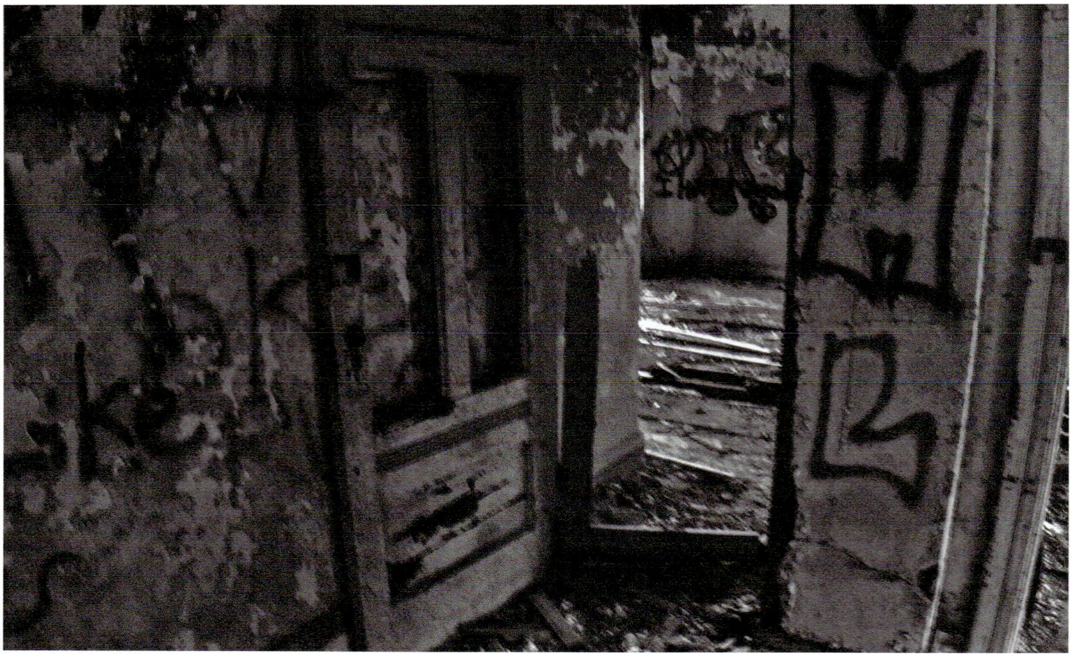

Most treated men came from training camps and not combat during the short months of operation, until the facility closed in 1919 and Hospital #26 would take over operating for sixteen months to help veterans become normal civilians again. (Jackson, 2010) *[Photo by Brian Cray]*

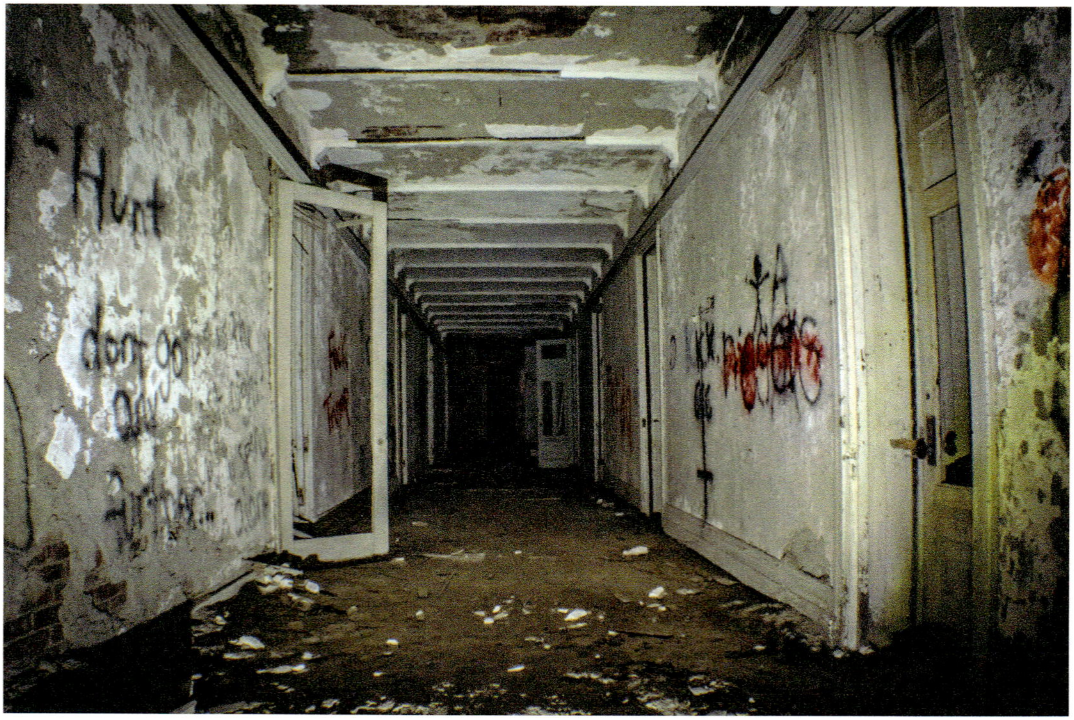

Those eerie nights of me wandering her halls felt as scary as they looked. *[Photo by Brian Cray]*

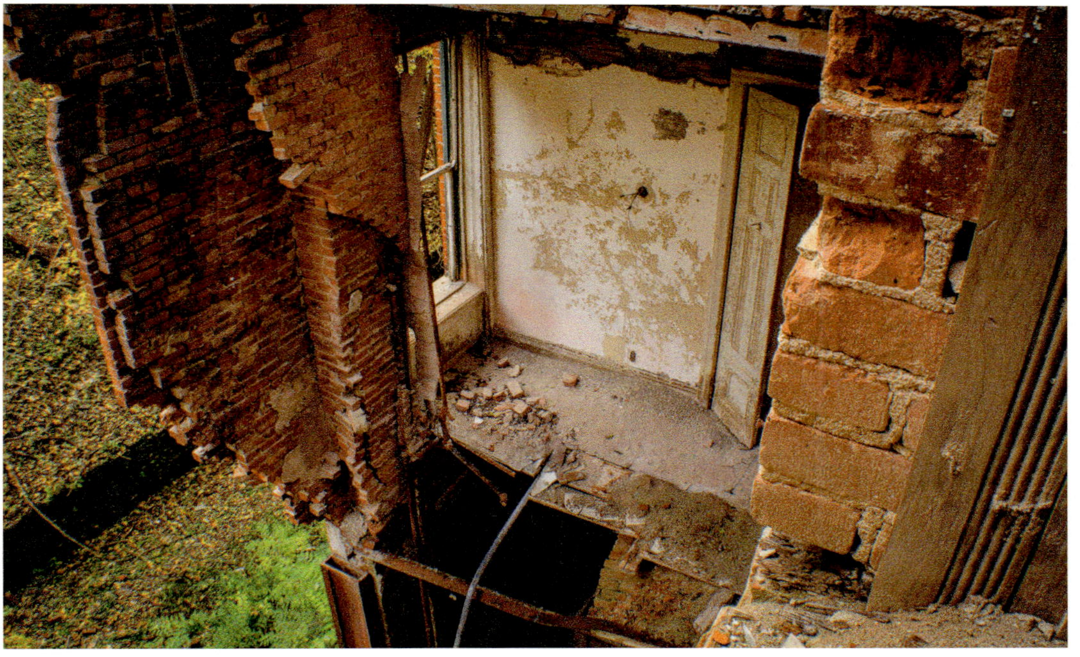

My feet tremble by the crumbling ledge of a door leading to nowhere. As my heart thumps, my eyes follow the sheared brick façade and focus on the empty room mangled by time, layered in grit and dust. There is something mystical about this moment, about this beautiful decay. *[Photo by Brian Cray]*

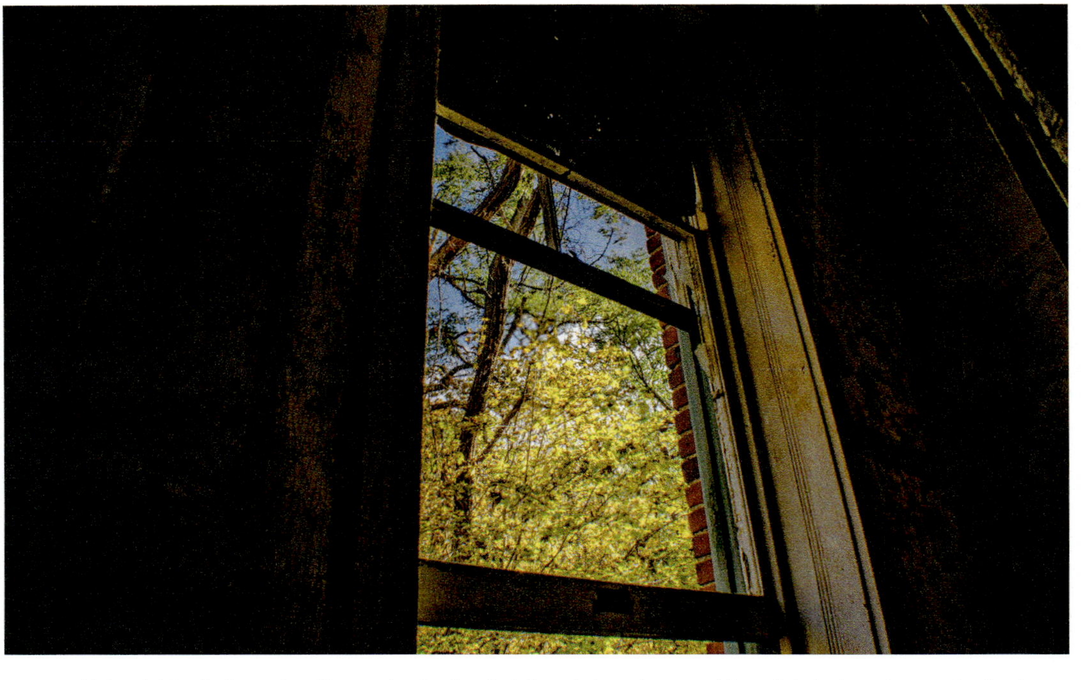

Light trickles in from the vibrant sky, for the first time in two days, and I can't help but stare at the luminous chartreuse forest. Through the blotch of leaves, the wiry branches encroach on the castle and soon they will engorge her rubble. *[Photo by Brian Cray]*

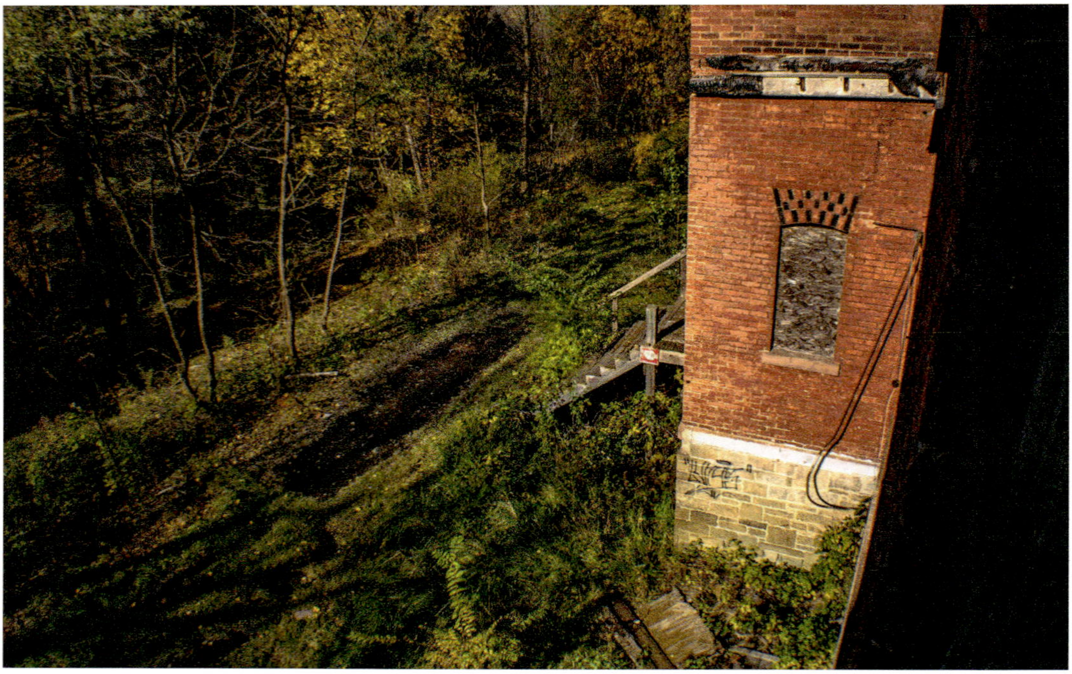

Checkered brick guides my eyes to a ribbed metal protrusion plastered along her fading crimson bones. I try to picture the wooden patio that once wrapped around her walls and guided guests above the front entrance, but there are no pieces left behind to finish the puzzle. *[Photo by Brian Cray]*

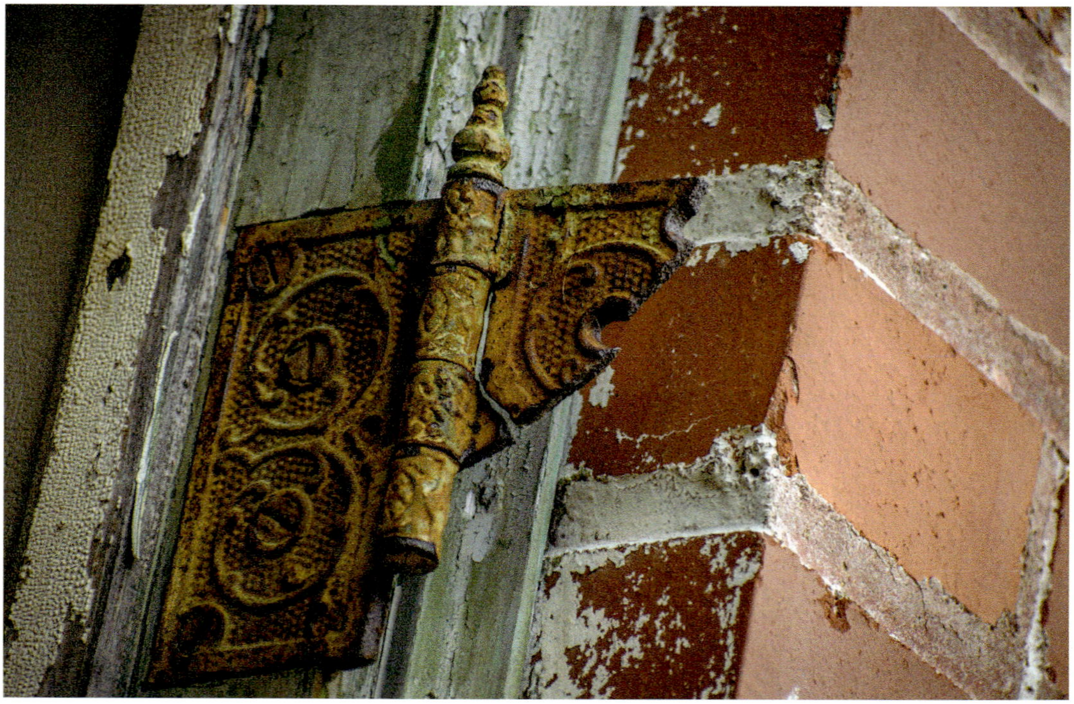

Hinges sheared from rust and rain paints the doors between their frames. *[Photo by Brian Cray]*

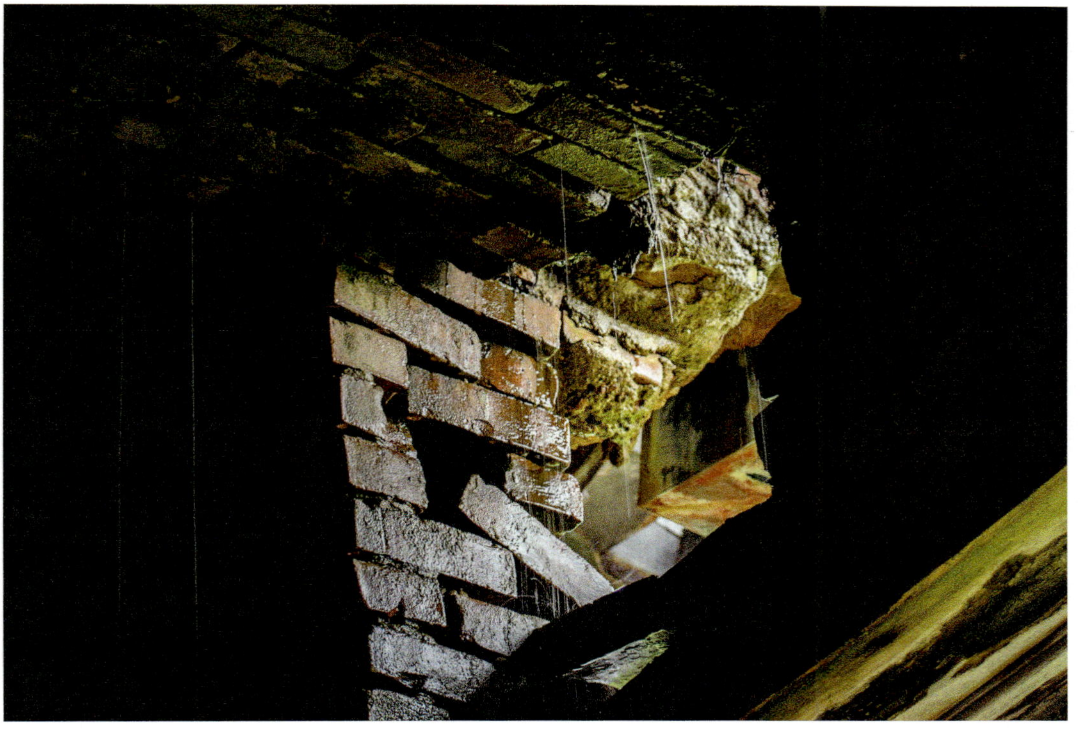

Smeared raindrops flood between the cracks of loose bricks in a frenzy of agonizing decay. *[Photo by Brian Cray]*

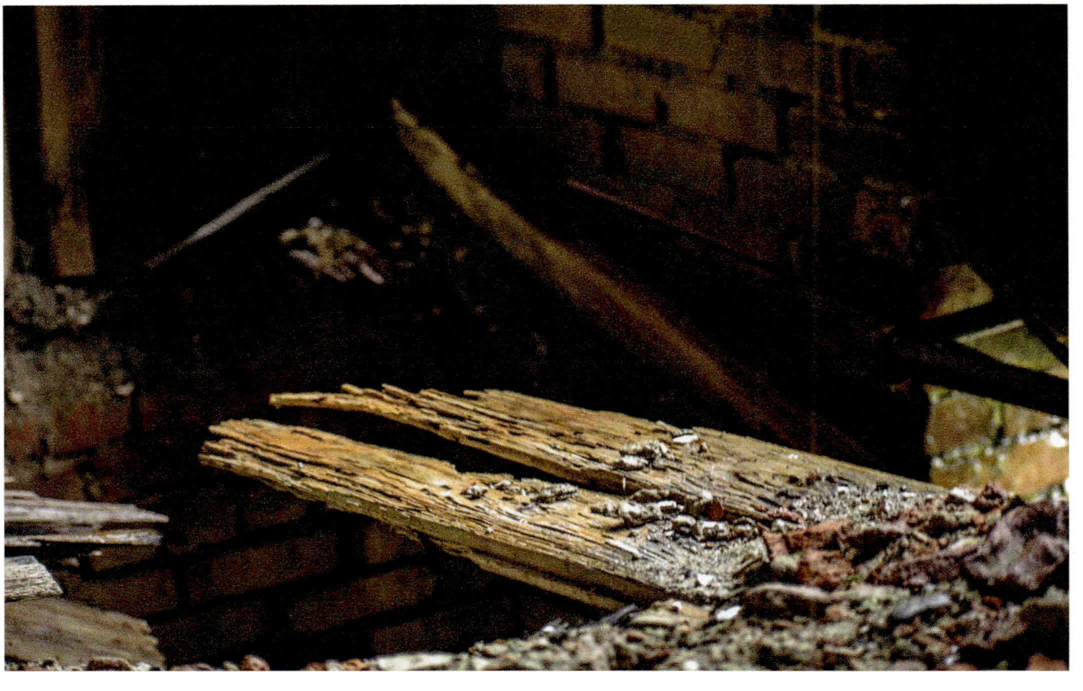

Beneath this splintered plank of oak, stray pebbles of debris plunge to the ground floor, contributing to her scars of decay. *[Photo by Brian Cray]*

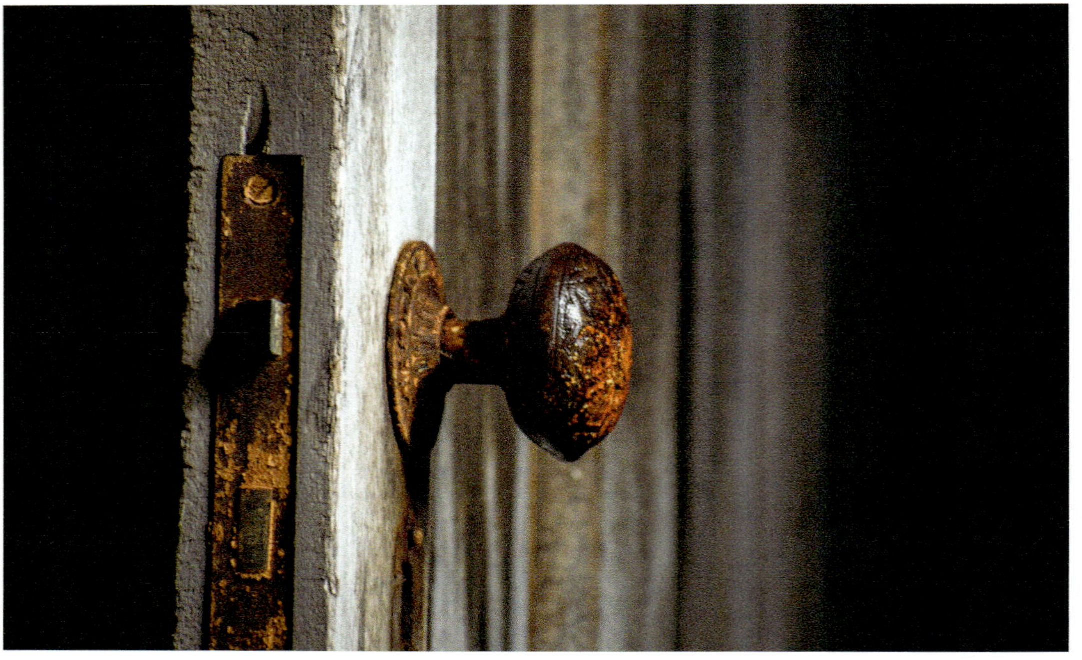

A river runs through every crack, down every brick, doorknob, and grain of wood when she compromised her roof to the lesions of winter. She will die a slow death, not by choice, but neglect. *[Photo by Brian Cray]*

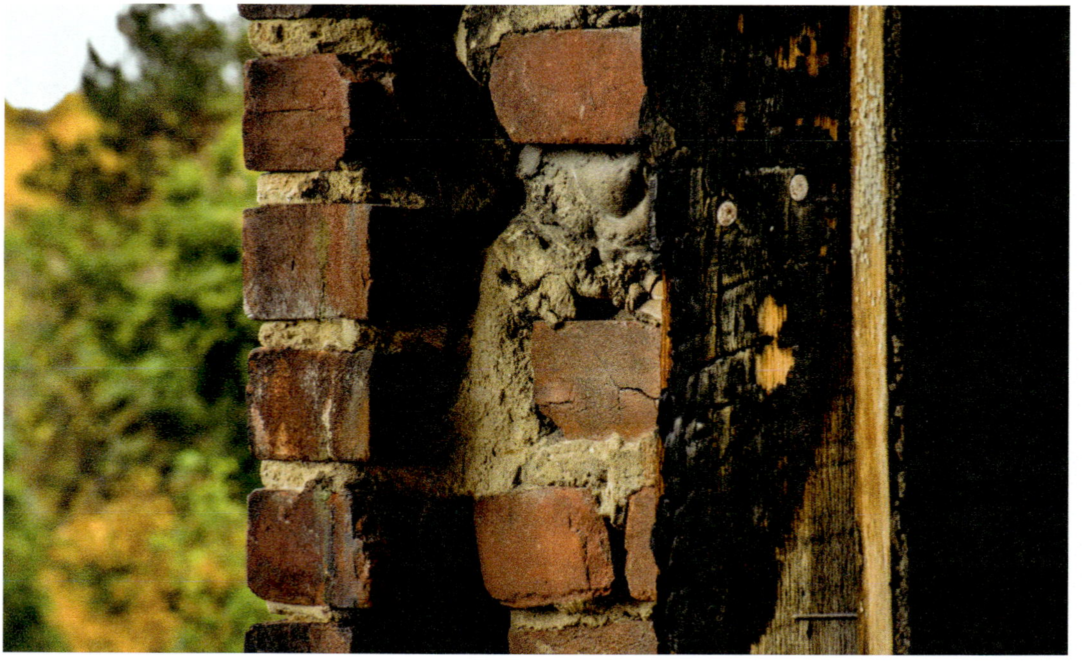

Charred wood demonstrates a series of arson attempts she has suffered throughout her years of neglect. Many of the cottages also no longer exist because of arsonists and trespassers not respecting the historical treasure that lurks on the hill. *[Photo by Brian Cray]*

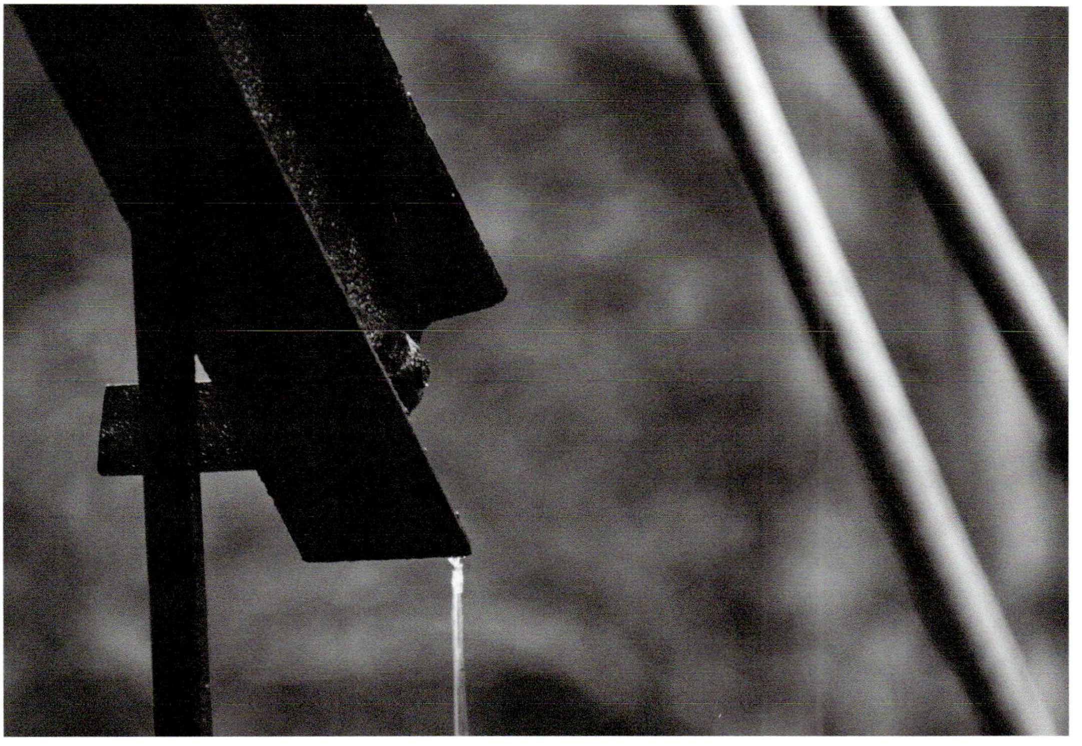

Above: Ramshackle steel beams act as water slides with warped metal pipes loosely dangling above. This marvel once supported 160 patients with another forty occupying the cottages spread along the hill. By the early 1900s, brochures stated patient capacity held 300 patrons. (Jackson, 2010) *[Photo by Brian Cray]*

Right: After nearly forty years of abandonment, her iron, her stone and her bricks still stand tall. Upon the construction of the new building in 1882, supporting walls were three to four feet in thickness and she stood upon twenty-seven piers as deep as ten feet. (Jackson, 2010) *[Photo by Brian Cray]*

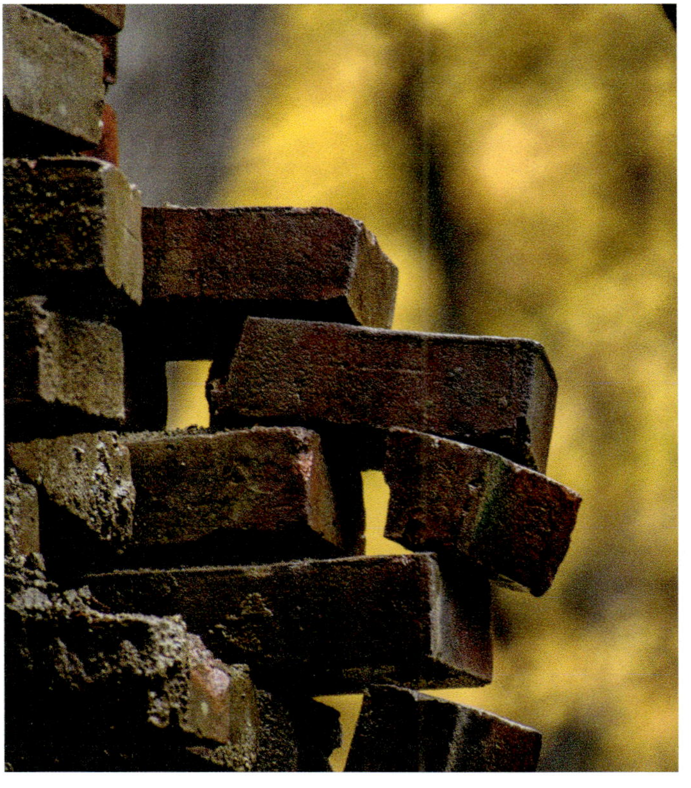

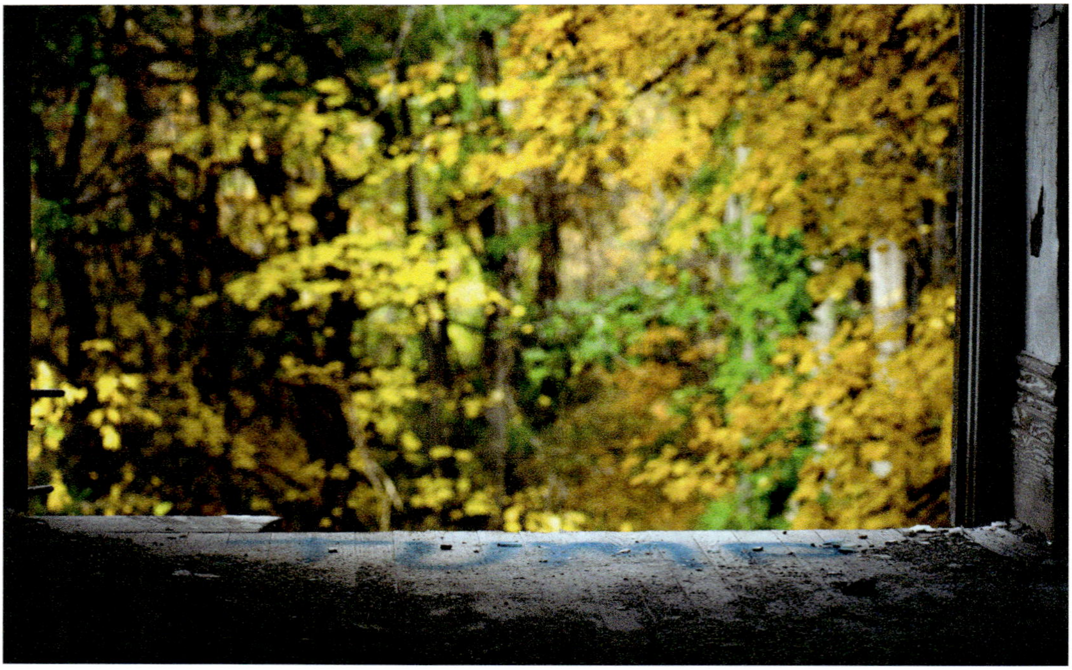

JUMP if you will, but the Olympic-size pool is far from the ledge. It's beyond the yellow and green blurs of forest, nestled in the lower woods. *[Photo by Brian Cray]*

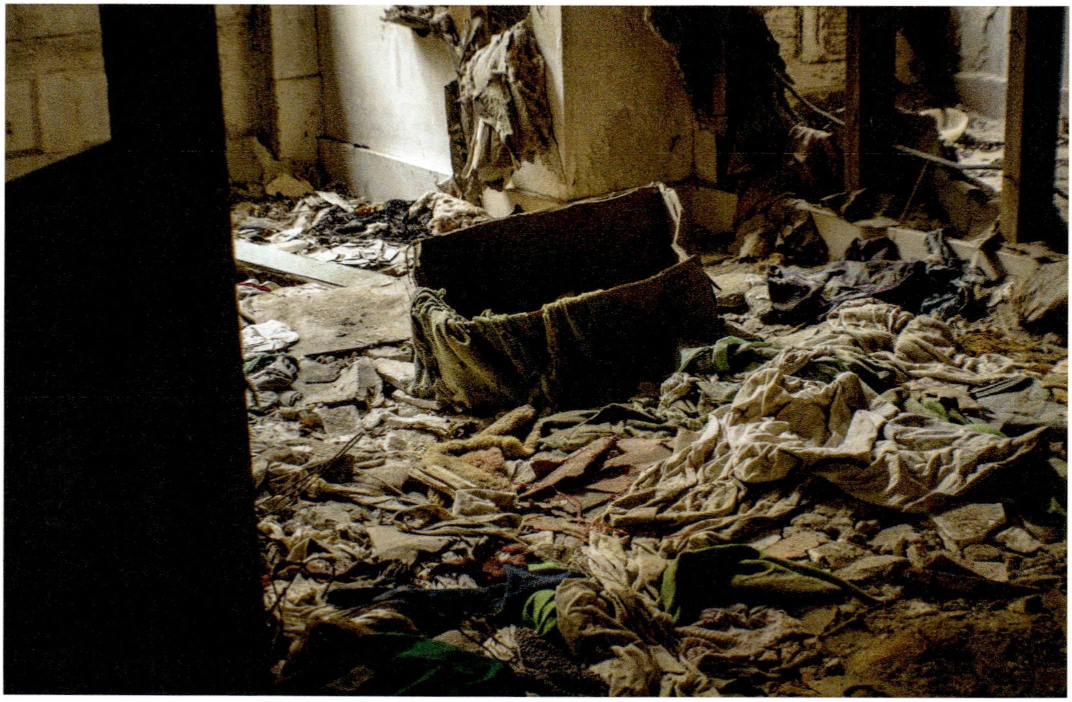

This is the only room in the main building was soiled with dirty laundry, which I found quite odd being that the basement, which is no longer accessible, contained the laundry room. (Jackson, 2010) *[Photo by Brian Cray]*

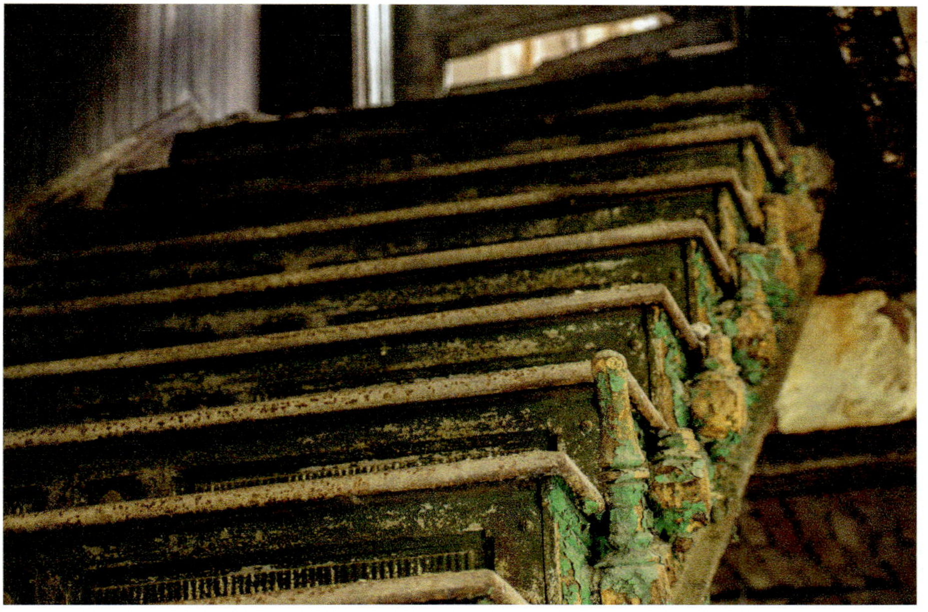

These green stairs lead to the third floor, where much of the same facilities existed for women along with more lodging rooms for patients. (Jackson, 2010) *[Photo by Brian Cray]*

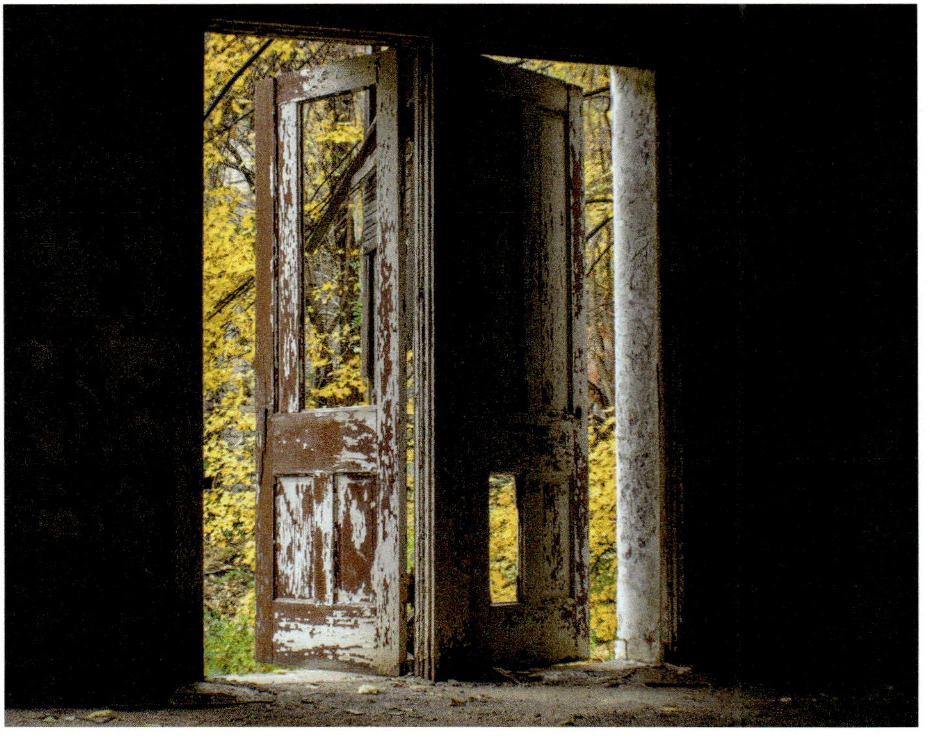

Two doors, left ajar, creak with the subtle gusting of wind, and beneath the chartreuse branches of autumn, lay heaps of brick and debris. Somewhere in this chaos, Moliere-Thermo-Electric, Russian, Electric and Leg Bath Rooms once existed. (Jackson, 2010) *[Photo by Brian Cray]*

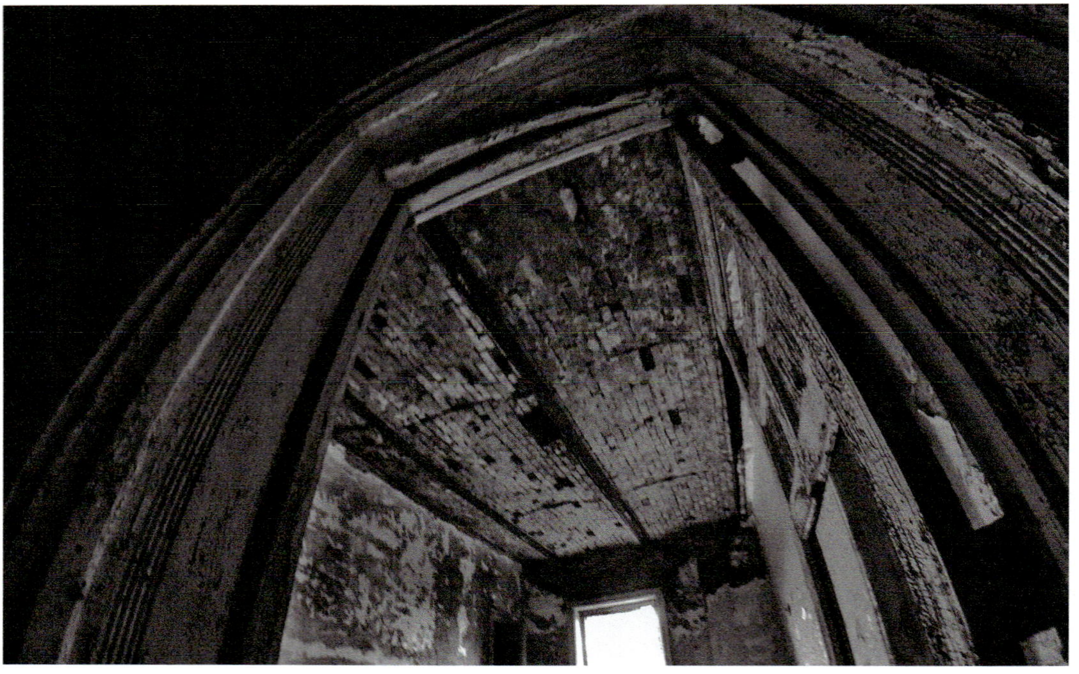

The second floor of the new building was mainly full of treatment facilities for men. This small room was most probably a shampooing room for Turkish Baths based on the diagram on page 65 of Ted Jackson's book *The Castles on the Hill. [Photo by Brian Cray]*

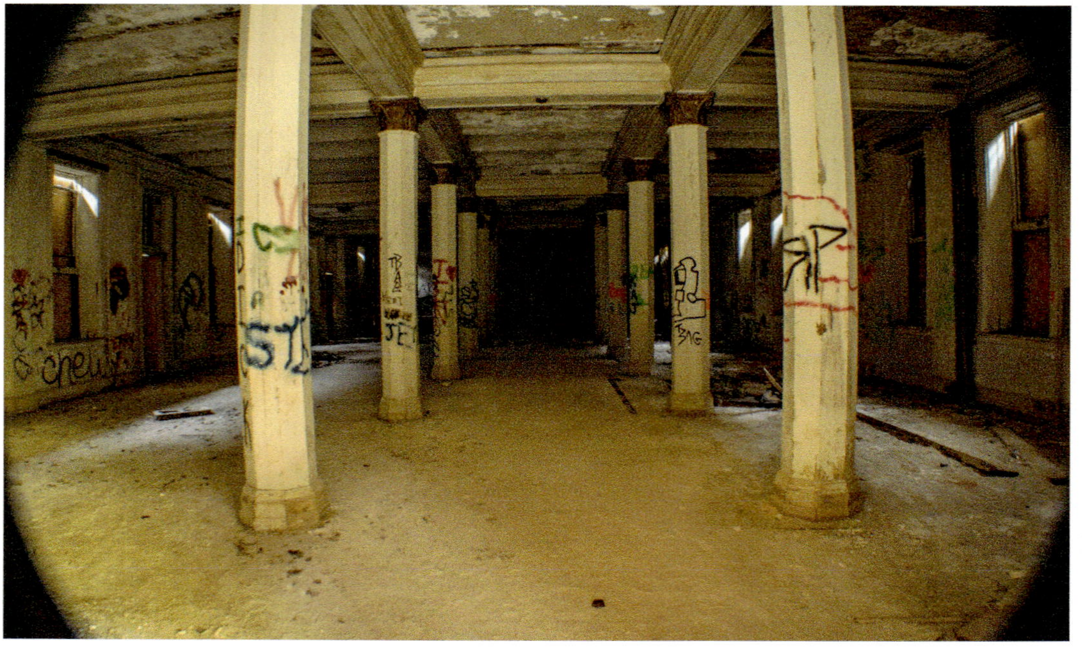

Light trickles in through the loose boards covering the windows to the old dining room. In the years following the fire, little changed with daily routine; however, a third optional meal was implemented, supper. (Jackson, 2010) *[Photo by Brian Cray]*

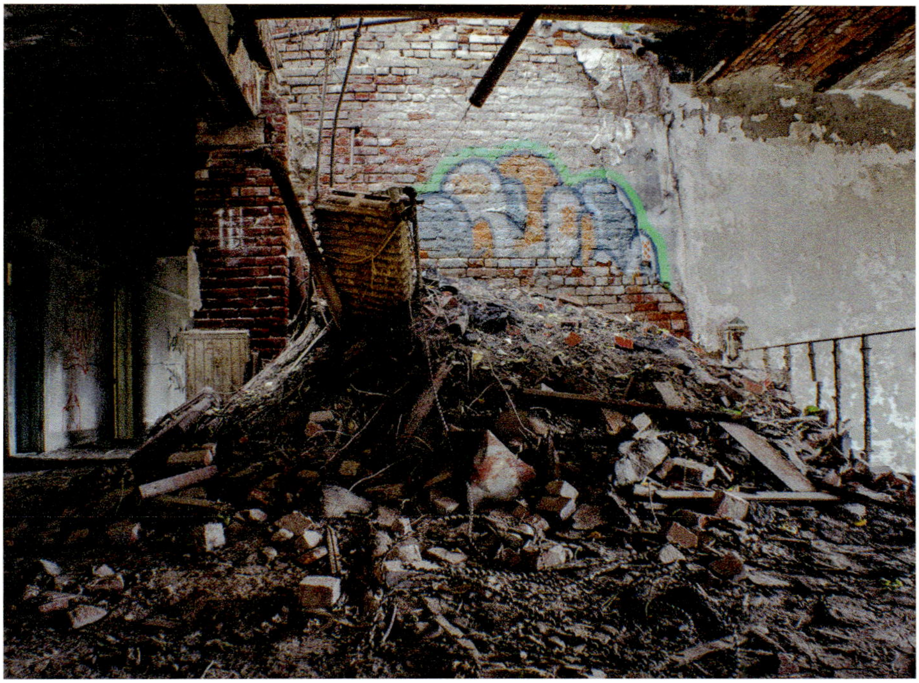

As we trek closer to the rooftop, it looks less structurally stable with mounds of debris piled high in corners along the wall where ceilings caved inward from years of repeated snow loads. Dansville is said to have the coldest and harshest winters of any city in Western New York. This is proof of the damage accompanied by winter's chilling breath. *[Photo by Brian Cray]*

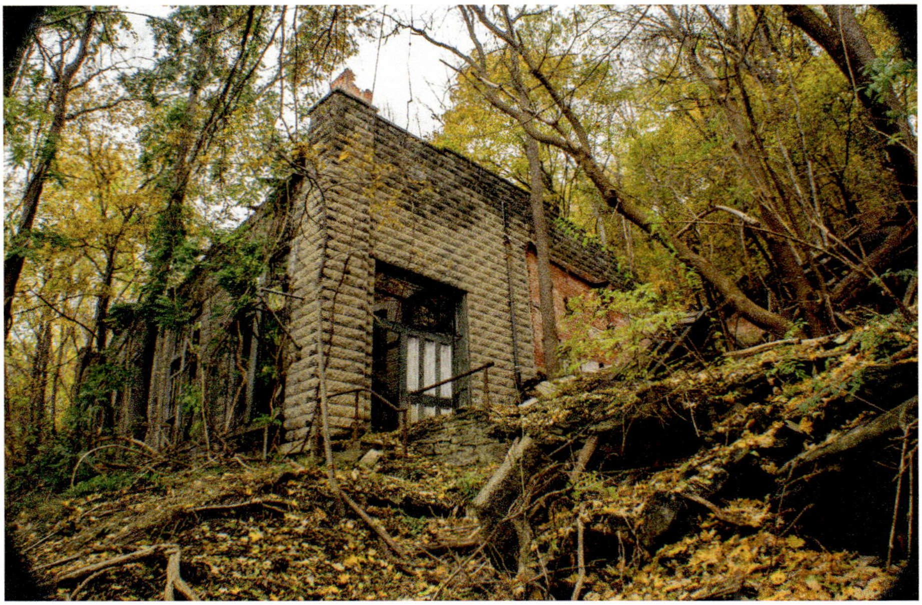

The powerhouse shown here provided the San with its own electrical services by the 1890s and along with it, forty more acres of land were purchased for cottages and farming to produce its own food over the years. (Jackson, 2010) *[Photo by Brian Cray]*

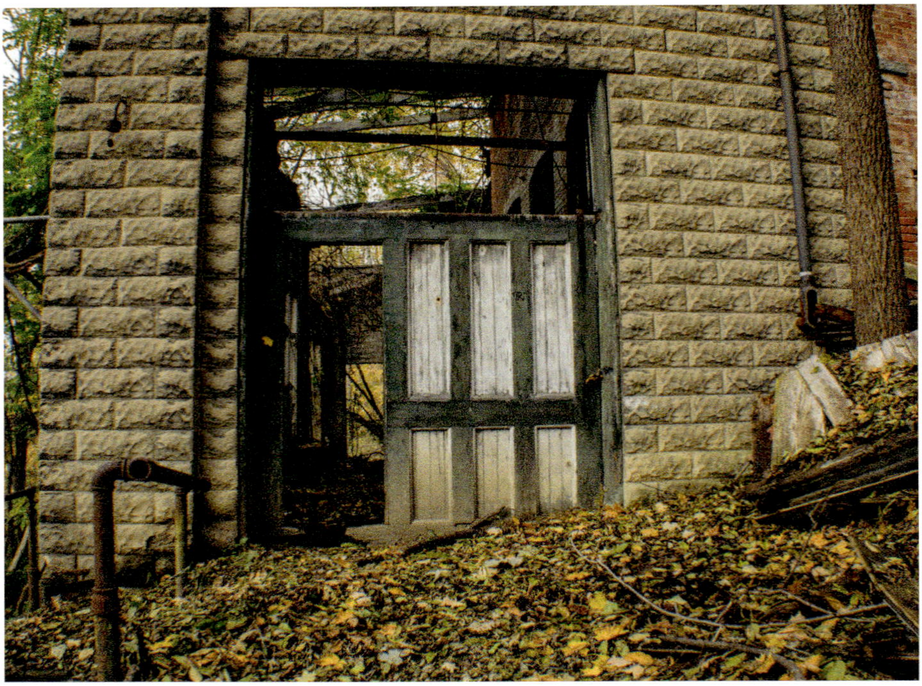

With the new powerhouse, the elevator no longer needed manual cranking, which made it easier for guests to get floor-to-floor, as well as help with business operations, especially for delivering freight (Jackson, 2010). *[Photo by Brian Cray]*

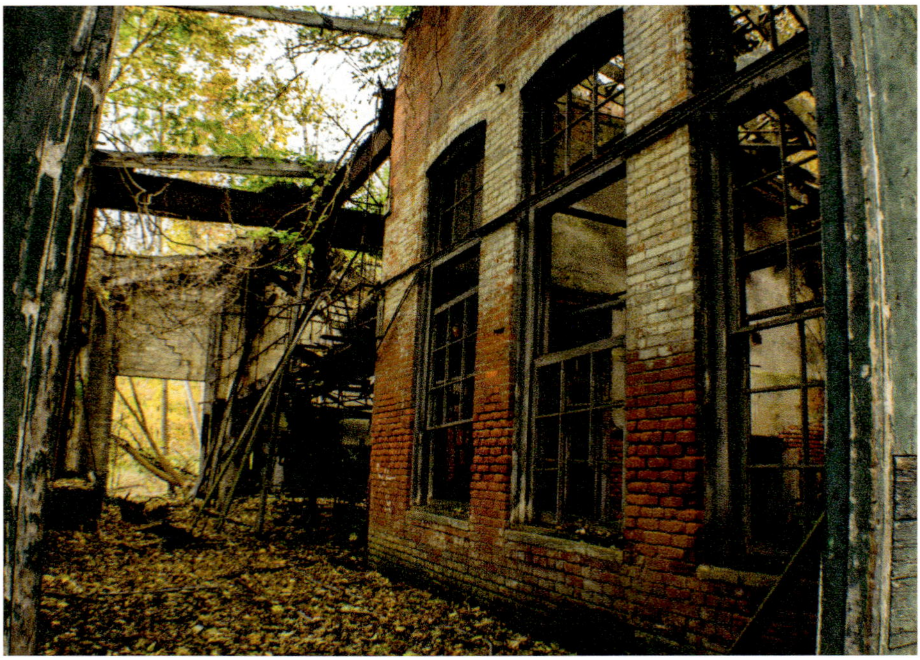

As I wander into the powerhouse, I focus on the bricks bleeding bright red, and my eyes shift to the open roof, scattered in chaos amidst the floor. *[Photo by Brian Cray]*

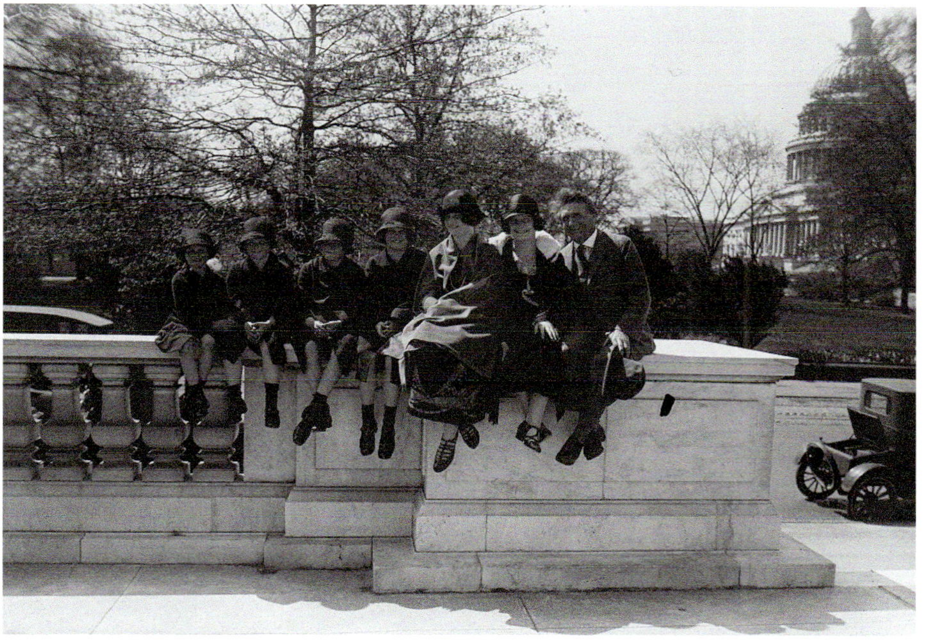

Another picture of Bernarr Macfadden in the spotlight with his family at the Capitol. Here he demonstrated how to keep fit to legislators. Left to right we have Beverly, Brannda, Benlah, Byrice, Helen, Byrne, and Bernarr. *[Photo by Harris & Ewing, photographer]*

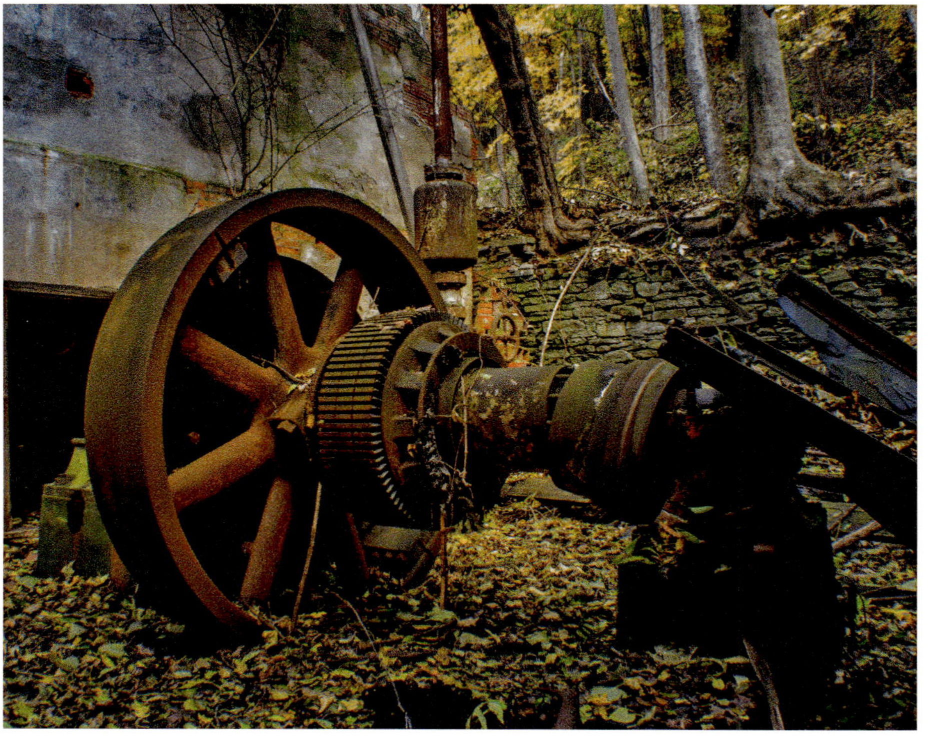

Gears afflicted by the concept of time aren't going anywhere soon. *[Photo by Brian Cray]*

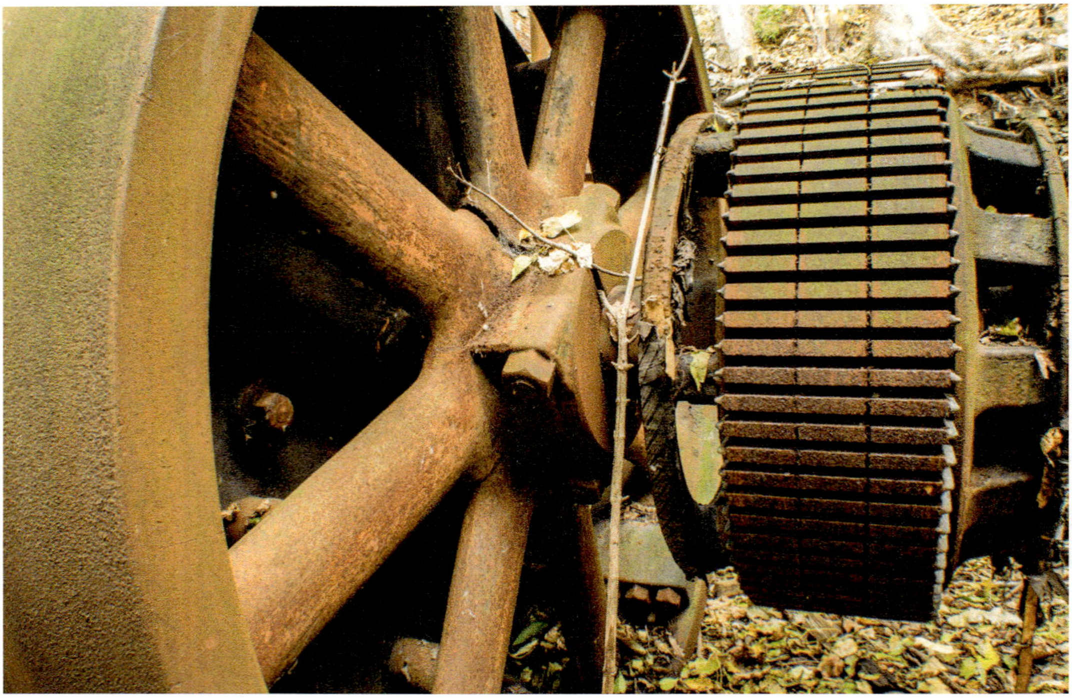

The wheels of time crank regardless of man's plans ... here's the bitter rusted iron(y). *[Photo by Brian Cray]*

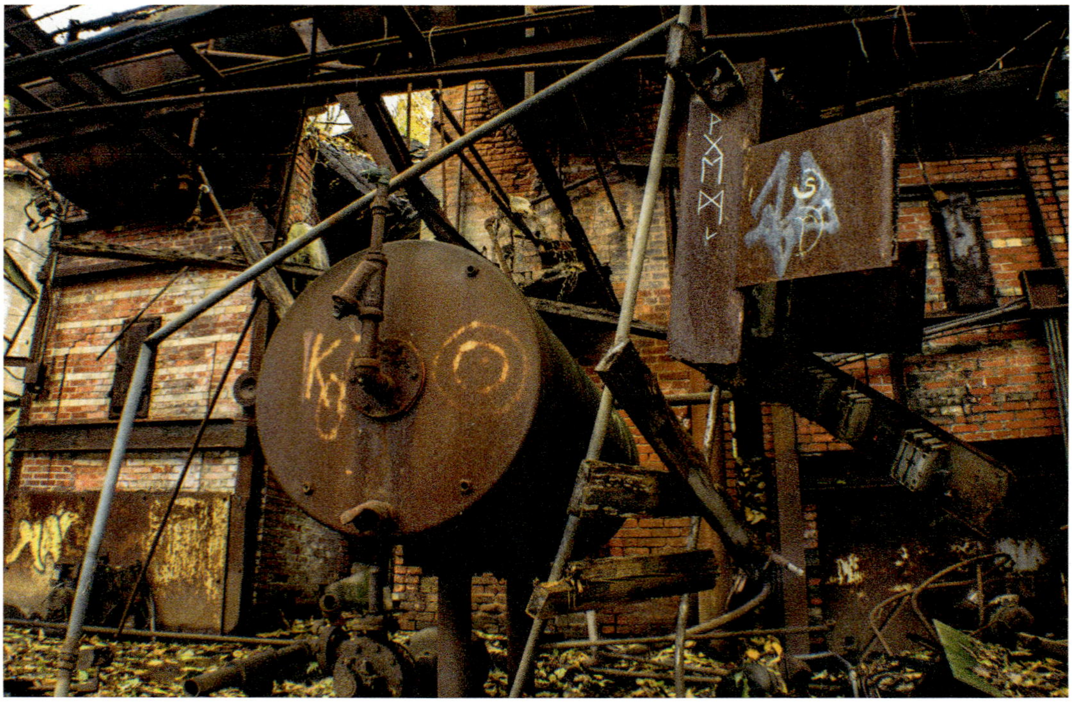

Rusted nuts, bolts and ramshackle pipes fester under ominous clouds. Through this pandemonium, the soft pitter of water and rustling of leaves soothes my ears as I listen to the sound of beautiful decay. *[Photo by Brian Cray]*

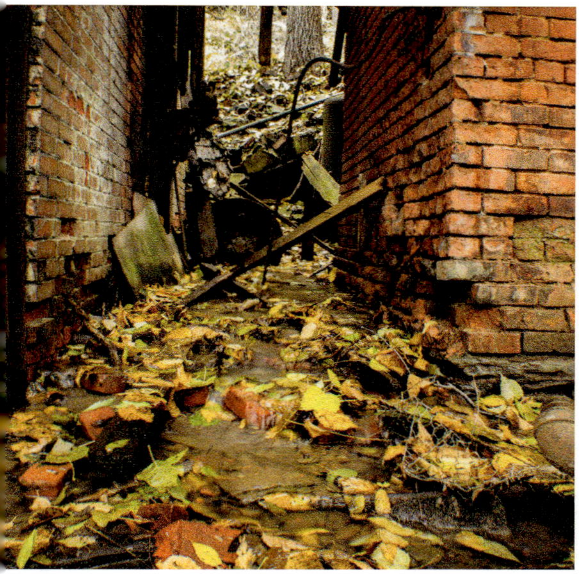

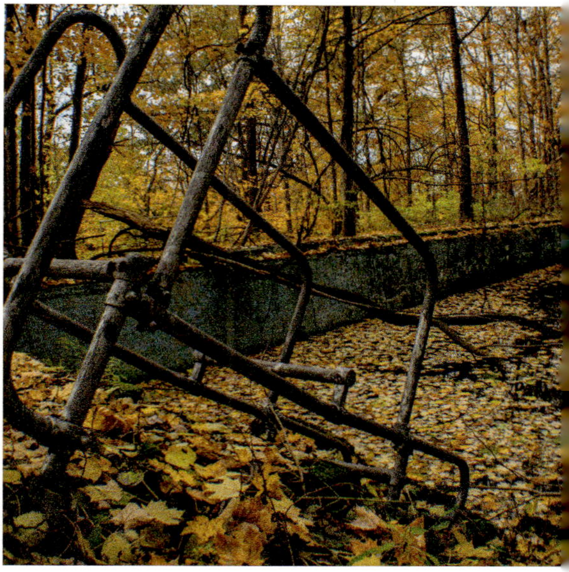

Above left: Water flows down the east hill like a river, running rampant through derelict corridors, bringing rusted gears, loose pipes, bricks, rubble, dead leaves, and anything in its path. *[Photo by Brian Cray]*

Above right: The pool no longer attracts mischievous kids sneaking into the P.C. at night or paying patrons, but sits as a shell of its past, canvassed in leaves and a black cauldron of hopelessness. *[Photo by Brian Cray]*

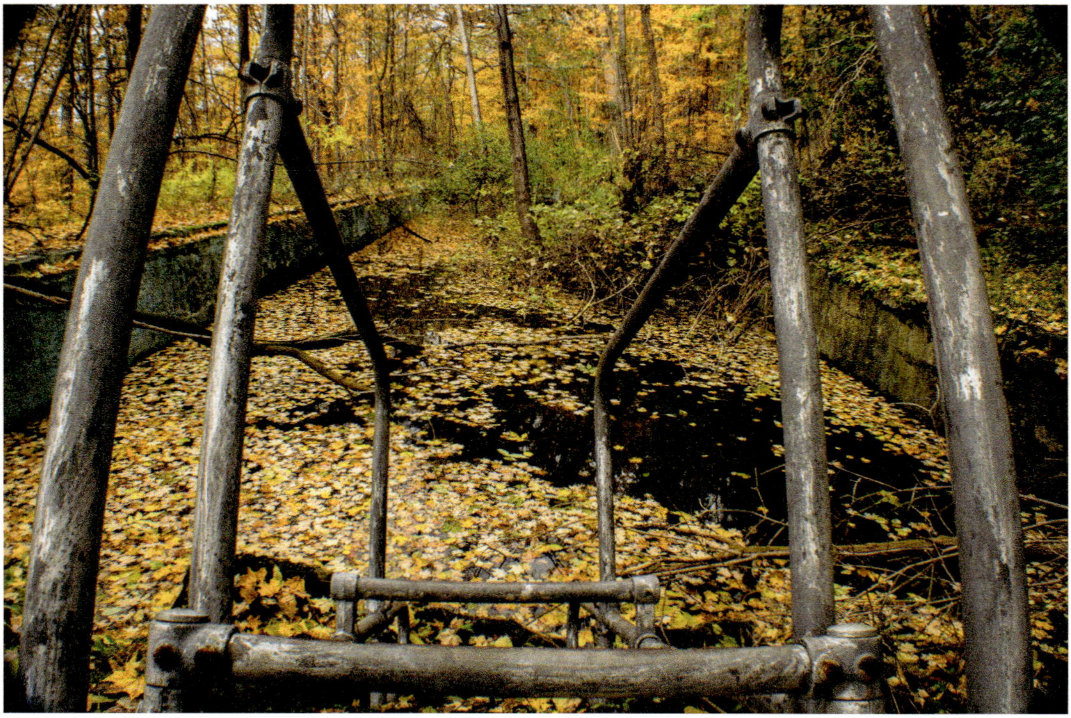

As I look out into the black lagoon, it feels endless in size and vast in memories. I have never seen a pool so extraordinary in size in all of my travels. *[Photo by Brian Cray]*

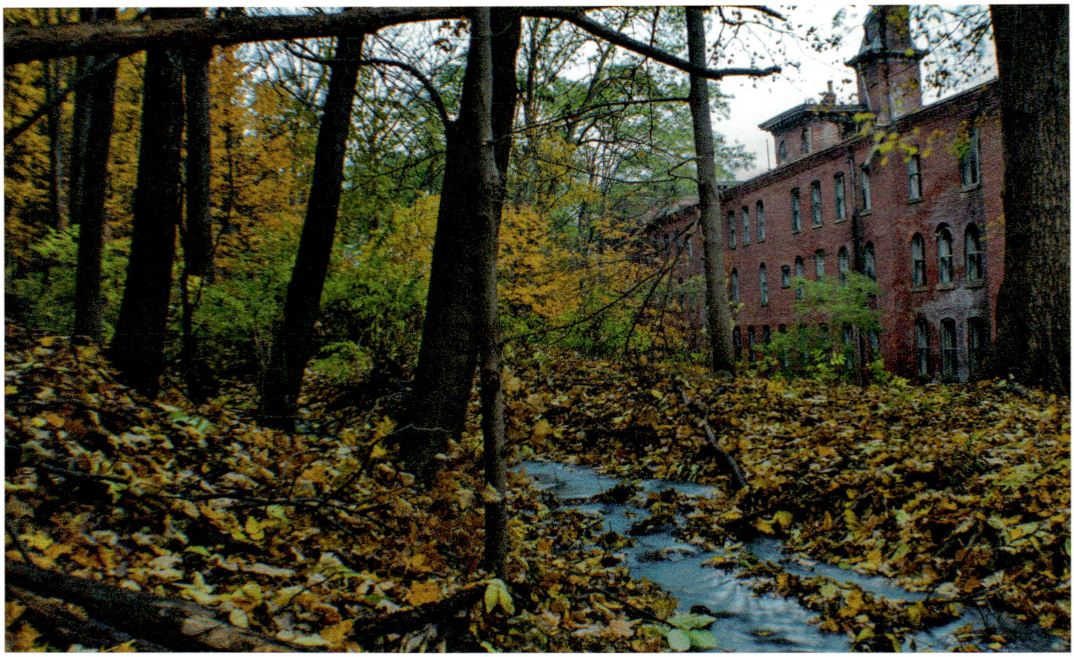

From the sun falling along the horizon, this low-light flick of the creek cascading along the east hill almost looks surreal. The still blue ripples guide my eyes to the red façade of castle standing tall through the decadence of trees and autumn leaves. *[Photo by Brian Cray]*

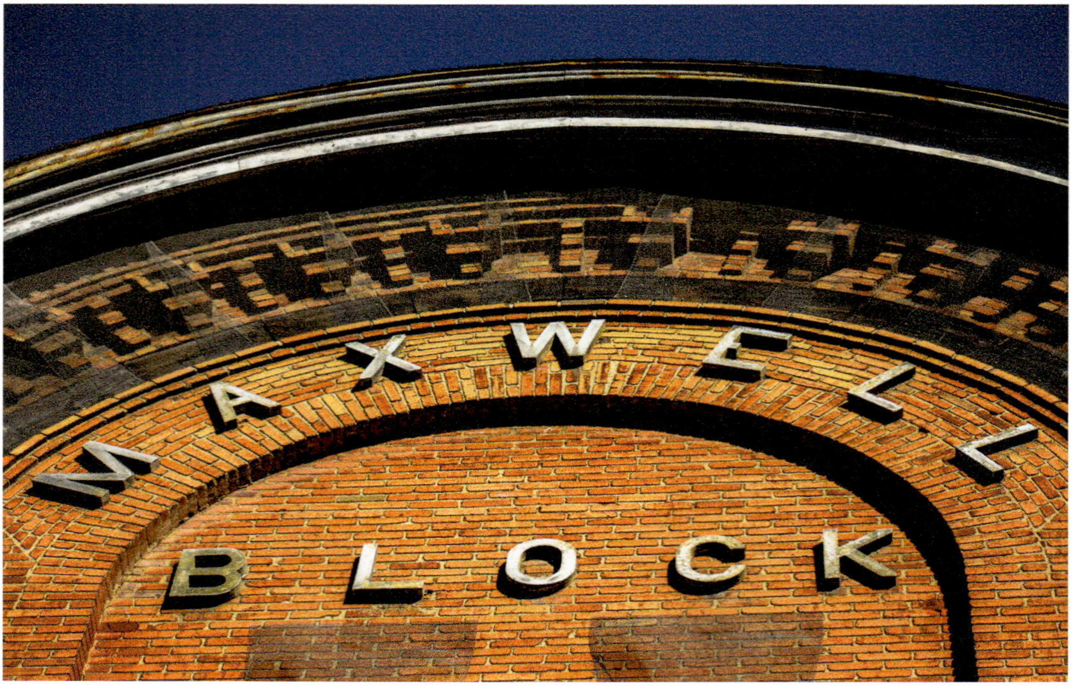

As I wander from the old Sugar Bowl Café, I stop as my eyes catch the attention of Maxwell Block. The red façade towers to the sky much like the construction of "the San." *[Photo by Brian Cray]*

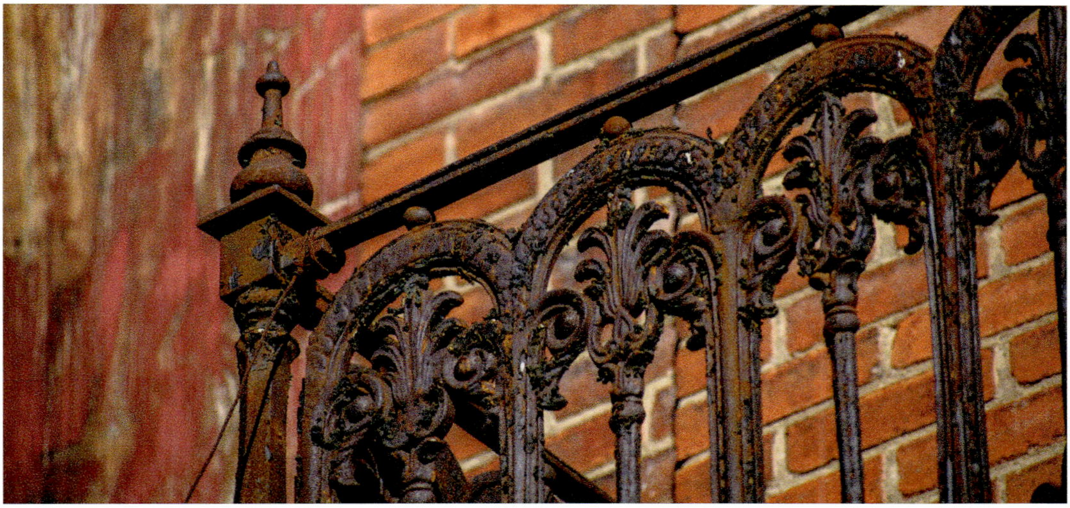

These balconies along the Maxwell Block of Main Street resemble those decaying at the San with slightly different intricacies in their designs. *[Photo by Brian Cray]*

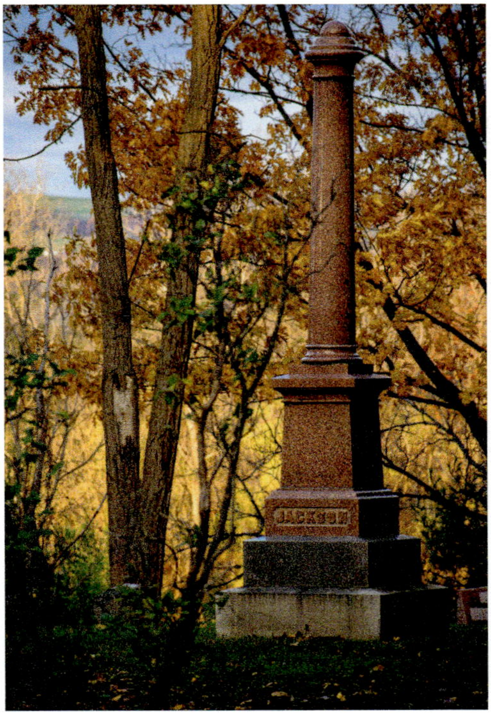

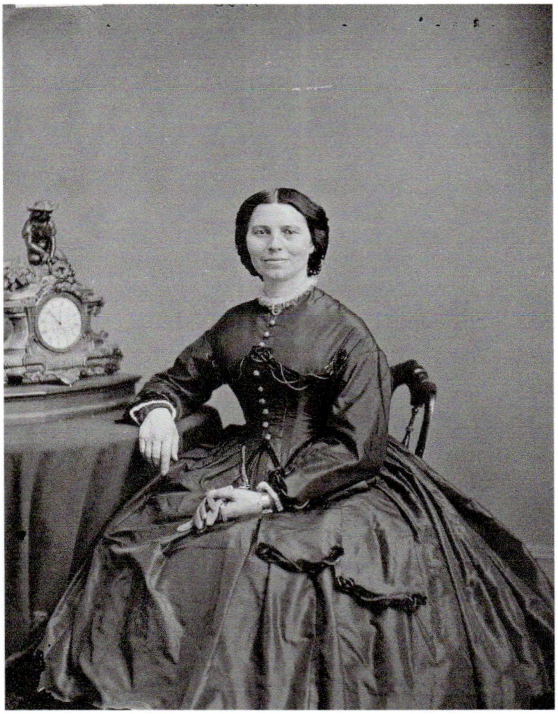

Above left: Jackson was diagnosed with cancer and moved to Berkshire Hills Sanitarium in North Adams, MA, for treatment. On a visit back to his home at Brightside cottage in Dansville, he died on July 11, 1895, and was buried in Green Mount Cemetery. (Jackson, 2010) *[Photo by Brian Cray]*

Above right: Clara Barton was a patient in 1876 and enjoyed the San so much that she rented a house in Dansville for ten years. She started the first chapter of the American Red Cross on August 22, 1881, in Dansville. (Jackson, 2010) *[Photo by Matthew Brady]*

ENDNOTES

Chapter 1

1. "Livingston County, New York," 2018
2. "Dansville"
3. Jackson, 2010
4. Bunnell & Quick, 1902
5. Fanelli, 2015
6. Gilbert, 2017
7. Fanelli, 2015
8. Jackson, 2010
9. Ibid
10. Ibid
11. Gilbert, 2017
12. Ibid
13. Kirsch, 2010
14. Ibid
15. Ibid
16. Ibid
17. "Bernarr Macfadden," 2018
18. Bennett, "Bernarr Macfadden, the Father of Physical Culture"
19. Adams, 2010
20. "Physical Culture Hotel," 1926
21. Kirsch, 2010
22. Gilbert, 2017
23. Adams, 2010
24. Bennett, "The Final Seven Years"

25. ibid
26. ibid
27. Gilbert, 2017
28. Jackson, 2010
29. ibid
30. ibid

Chapter 2

1. Bunnell & Quick, 1902
2. ibid
3. ibid
4. ibid
5. ibid
6. ibid
7. Jackson, 2010
8. ibid
9. Carson, 1957
10. Jackson, 2010
11. ibid
12. ibid
13. Carson, 1957
14. Jackson, 2010
15. "Dress Reform"
16. Jackson, 2010
17. Carson, 1957
18. Jackson, 2010
19. ibid
20. Bunnell & Quick, 1902
21. *Year book of the Jackson Sanatorium, Dansville, N.Y.: 1898*, 1899
22. Carson, 1957
23. Jackson & Austin, 1869, pp. 305
24. ibid
25. ibid
26. "Dress Reform"
27. Jackson & Austin, 1869, pp. 305
28. Jackson, 1916, pp. 3
29. Bunnell & Quick, 1902
30. Gratzer, 2005
31. ibid
32. ibid
33. ibid

34. ibid
35. ibid
36. Chavey
37. Carson, 1957
38. ibid
39. ibid
40. Bunnell & Quick, 1902
41. Jackson, 2010
42. ibid
43. Jackson, 1916, pp. 19
44. Jackson, 1916, pp. 22
45. Cook & Huynh, 2006
46. ibid
47. Jackson, 2010

Chapter 3

1. This historical fiction adaptation was based off the diary of Elizabeth Walker's stay at "Our Home" in 1861-1862 from Ted Jackson's book *The Castles on the Hill*. I filled in the gaps with imagery from my multiple visits to Dansville over the years along with compiling several days of her stay into one, loosely based on "Our Home's" summer schedule to paint the picture of a typical day. For more firsthand accounts of the 1860s, refer to Ted Jackson's *The Castles on the Hill* and for a better description of life in the sanatorium beyond the 1860s refer to William Conklin's *The Jackson Health Resort*, if you are lucky enough to find a copy of it. I was not (limited copies available for the public according to Ted Jackson).

Chapter 4

1. Jackson, 2010
2. Wood, 2010
3. Adams, 2010
4. Ernst, 1991
5. Adams, 2010
6. Ernst, 1991
7. ibid
8. Adams, 2010
9. Ernst, 1991
10. ibid
11. Adams, 2010
12. Wood, 2010

13. ibid
14. Ernst, 1991
15. ibid
16. Adams, 2010
17. ibid
18. ibid
19. Ernst, 1991
20. Adams, 2010
21. ibid
22. ibid
23. ibid
24. Ernst, 1991
25. Adams, 2010
26. ibid
27. ibid
28. ibid
29. Ernst, 1991
30. ibid
31. Adams, 2010
32. ibid
33. ibid
34. Adams, 2010
35. Ernst, 1991
36. Adams, 2010
37. ibid
38. ibid
39. ibid
40. ibid
41. ibid
42. ibid
43. Mrozek, 1987
44. Adams, 2010
45. ibid
46. ibid
47. ibid
48. ibid
49. ibid
50. ibid
51. "Physical Culture Hotel," 1926
52. ibid
53. Ernst, 1991
54. "Physical Culture Hotel"
55. Adams, 2010

56. Ernst, 1991
57. ibid
58. ibid
59. "Physical Culture Hotel," 1926
60. ibid
61. Adams, 2010
62. ibid
63. ibid

CHAPTER 5

1. Adams, 2010
2. Mrozek, 1987
3. ibid
4. Adams, 2010
5. Gratzer, 2005
6. Adams, 2010
7. "Bernarr Macfadden," 2018
8. Adams, 2010
9. ibid
10. Bennett, "Bernarr Macfadden, the Father of Physical Culture"
11. Black, 2013
12. "Seven to Save – 2001"
13. Baker, 2016

BIBLIOGRAPHY

TEXT

26 Killed When Fast Train, Trying to Make Up Time, Is Wrecked. (1943, August 31). *The News-Herald*, p. 6. Retrieved February 12, 2019, from https://www.newspapers.com/clip/2690798/wayland_ny_aug_31_1943_uptrain/

Adams, M. (2010). *Mr. America: How Muscular Millionaire Bernarr Macfadden Transformed the Nation Through Sex, Salad, and the Ultimate Starvation Diet.* United States: It Books

Arnold, W. (2009, November 22). The Castle on the Hill - Jackson Sanatorium. Retrieved November 17, 2018, from https://www.artofabandonment.com/2009/11/the-castle-on-the-hill-jackson-sanatorium-10-16-2009/

Baker, C. (2016, May 16). Trespassing Spikes at Dansville's Abandoned 'Castle on the Hill'. Retrieved November 17, 2018, from https://geneseesun.com/trespassing-spikes-at-dansvilles-abandoned-castle-on-the-hill/

Bennett, J. M. (n.d.). Bernarr Macfadden - the Father of Physical Culture. Retrieved November 17, 2018, from http://www.bernarrmacfadden. com/

Bennett, J. M. (n.d.). The Final Seven Years. Retrieved November 18, 2018, from http://www.bernarrmacfadden.com/macfadden7.html

Bernarr Macfadden. (1926). *Physical Culture Hotel* [Brochure]. Author. Retrieved November 17, 2018, from http://www.riverflow.com/macfadden/pchotelbrochure/index.html

Bernarr Macfadden. (2018, August 23). Retrieved November 17, 2018, from https://en.m.wikipedia.org/wiki/Bernarr_Macfadden

Black, A., M., & R. (Eds.). (2013, June 19). Jackson Sanatorium. Retrieved November 17, 2018, from https://www.atlasobscura.com/places/jackson-sanitarium

Carson, G. (1957) *Cornflake Crusade.* [New York, Rinehart & Company] [Pdf] Retrieved from the Library of Congress, https://www.loc.go/item/57009631/

Chavey, E. (n.d.). The Early Days Of Breakfast Cereal. (n.d.). Retrieved November 17, 2018, from https://www.mrbreakfast.com/article.asp?articleid=13

Cook, W. R., & Huynh, E. C. (2006). *Around Dansville.* Charleston, SC: Arcadia Pub

Dansville. (n.d.). Retrieved November 16, 2018, from https://twainsgeography.com/content/dansville

Dress Reform. (n.d.). Retrieved November 17, 2018, from https://freethought-trail.org/causes/cause:dress-reform/

Ernst, R. (1991). *Weakness is a crime: The Life of Bernarr Macfadden.* Syracuse, NY: Syracuse University Press

Fanelli, G. (2015, October 05). The Castle on the Hill: A Story of American Decay. Retrieved November 17, 2018, from https://reporter.rit.edu/leisure/castle-hill-story-american-decay

Gilbert, D. (2017, April 15). Castle on the Hill. Retrieved November 17, 2018, from https://dansvillelibrary.org/community/castle-on-the-hill/

Gratzer, W. B. (2005). *Terrors of the table: The curious history of nutrition.* Oxford: Oxford University Press. doi:http://lib1.org/_ads/979bbcb4a8bc5fa3fd4e4ca0c5405428

Jackson, J. C. (1871). *How to treat the sick without medicine.* Jackson, Austin & Company. doi: https://books.google.com Jackson, J. C., & Austin, H. N. (1869). *The Sexual Organism: And Its Healthful Management.* New York: B.Leverett Emerson. doi:https://books.google.com

Jackson, J. H. (1916). *The Jackson Health Resort: Dansville, Livingston County, New York: Health for All.* Geneseo, NY: Milne Library. Reprint

Jackson, T. (2010). *The Castles on the Hill.* Dansville, NY: Dansville Area Historical Society.

Kirsch, T. (2010, June 21). Jackson Sanatorium. Retrieved November 17, 2018, from https://opacity.us/site113_jackson_sanatorium.htm

Livingston County, New York. (2018, September 28). Retrieved November 17, 2018, from https://en.m.wikipedia.org/wiki/Dansville,_Livingston_County,_New_York

Mrozek, D. (1987). The Scientific Quest for Physical Culture and the Persistent Appeal of Quackery. *Journal of Sport History,* 14(1), 76-86. Retrieved from http://www.jstor.org/stable/43609327

Oursler, F. (n.d.) The Most Unforgettable Characters I've Met. Retrieved November 17, 2018, from http://www.riverflow.com/macfadden/mucim.html

Quick, F. I. (1902). *Dansville: Historical, Biographical, Descriptive* (A. O. Bunnell, Ed.). Dansville, NY: Instructor Publishing Company. doi: https://www.amazon.com/Dansville-historical-biographical-descriptive-Bunnell-ebook/dp/B00AH017N2/ref=mp_s_a_1_1?ie=UTF8&qid=1549921894&sr=1-1&pi=AC_SX236_SY340_FMwebp_QL65&keywords=dansville, historical&dpPl=1&dpID=41TCfZVLHQL&ref=plSrch

Raga, S. (2016, March 18). James Caleb Jackson, Inventor of Dry Breakfast

Cereal. Retrieved November 17, 2018, from http://mentalfloss.com/article/77286/retrobituaries-james-caleb-jackson-inventor-dry-breakfast-cereal

Seven to Save - 2001. (n.d.). Retrieved November 17, 2018, from https://www.preservenys.org/seven-to-save---2001.html

Wheeler, A. D. (2017, May 15). Jackson Sanatorium ~ Dansville, NY. Retrieved November 17, 2018, from https://www.theexplorographer.com/2012/02/our-castle-on-the-hill/

Wood, C. (1974). *Bernarr Macfadden: A Study in Success.* New York: Beekman

Year book of the Jackson Sanatorium, Dansville, N.Y.: 1898. (1899). Dansville, NY: Jackson Sanatorium

Photographs

Detroit Publishing Co, P. *Jackson Sanatorium, Dansville, N.Y.* Dansville Dansville. New York New York State United States, None. [Between 1890 and 1901] [Photograph] Retrieved from the Library of Congress, https://www.loc.gov/item/2016801269/

Sartain, Emily, photographer. *James Caleb Jackson.* [Photograph] Retrieved from the National Library Medicine, https://commons.m.wikimedia.org/wiki/File:James_Caleb_Jackson3.jpg

Bain News Service, P. *B. MacFadden.* [No Date Recorded on Caption Card] [Photograph] Retrieved from the Library of Congress, https://www.loc.gov/item/2014717467

Detroit Publishing Co, P. *Dansville, N.Y.* New York New York State United States, None. [Between 1890 and 1901] [Photograph] Retrieved from the Library of Congress, https://www.loc.gov/item/2016799384/

(*ca.* 1893*) Nude male, Prof. B.A. McFadden, full-length portrait, standing on pedestal, facing left, wearing a fig leaf, with hands behind head.* , ca. 1893. [Photograph] Retrieved from the Library of Congress, https://www.loc.gov/item/97510663/

Harris & Ewing, photographer. (1924) *Bernarr MacFadden, famous physical culture expert of N.Y. and Sen. Smith W. Brookhart of Iowa, staged a boxing match outside Sen. office bldg.* United States United States, 1924. [April] [Photograph] Retrieved from the Library of Congress, https://www.loc.gov/item/2016887215/

Harris & Ewing, photographer. (1932) *Group outside 1 Cent Restaurant, National Demonstration, Bernarr MacFadden Foundation Unemployment Relief.* United States United States, 1932. [or 1933] [Photograph] Retrieved from the Library of Congress, https://www.loc.gov/item/2016890054/

Harris & Ewing, photographer. (1924) *Bernarr MacFadden, famous physical culture expert, and his family, at the Capitol where they are demonstrating how to keep fit to the legislators. L. to r.: Beverly, Brannda, Benlah, Byrice, Helen, Byrne, and Mr. MacFadden.* District of Columbia United States Washington D.C. Washington D.C, 1924. [April] [Photograph]

Retrieved from the Library of Congress, https://www.loc.gov/item/2016887216/
Brady, Matthew, photographer. (1921-1940) *Miss Clara Barton* [Photograph] Retrieved from, https://catalog.archives.gov/id/526057

Fact captions are derived from Ted Jackson's book *The Castles on the Hill* and Mark Adams's book *Mr. America: How Muscular Millionaire Bernarr Macfadden Transformed the Nation Through Sex, Salad, and the Ultimate Starvation Diet.* Historical photos are in the public domain with sources listed in italic brackets and all other photos are copyright of Brian Cray.